6/8/96   ②

COLOUR YOU ATTRACTIVE

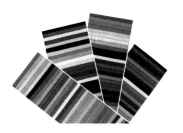

foulsham

LONDON • NEW YORK • TORONTO • SYDNEY

**Colours to suit your Clothes
your Jewellery • your Make-up
your Glasses • your Hair**

COLOU

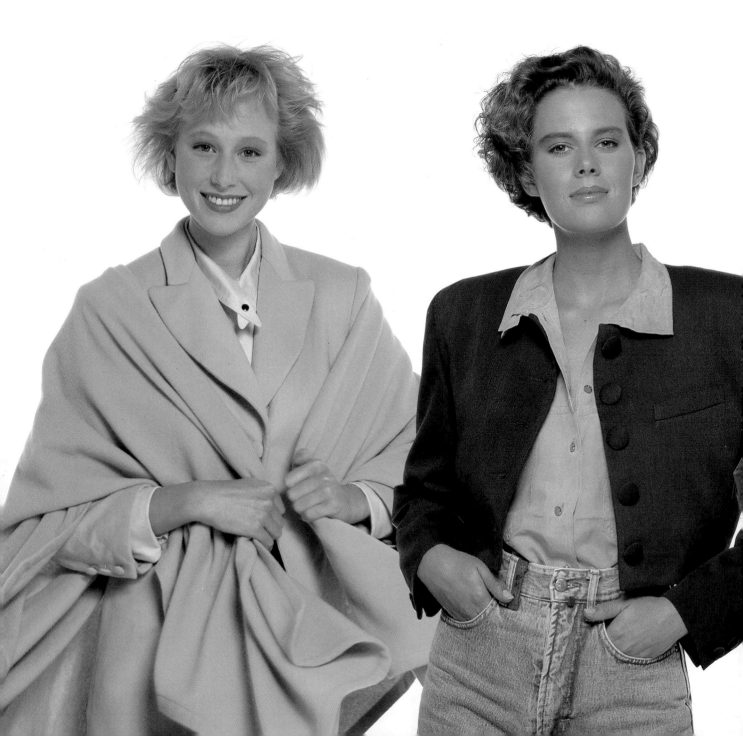

R **Y**OU **A**TTRACTIVE

by Christina Buscher

With 8 colour charts for colour type testing

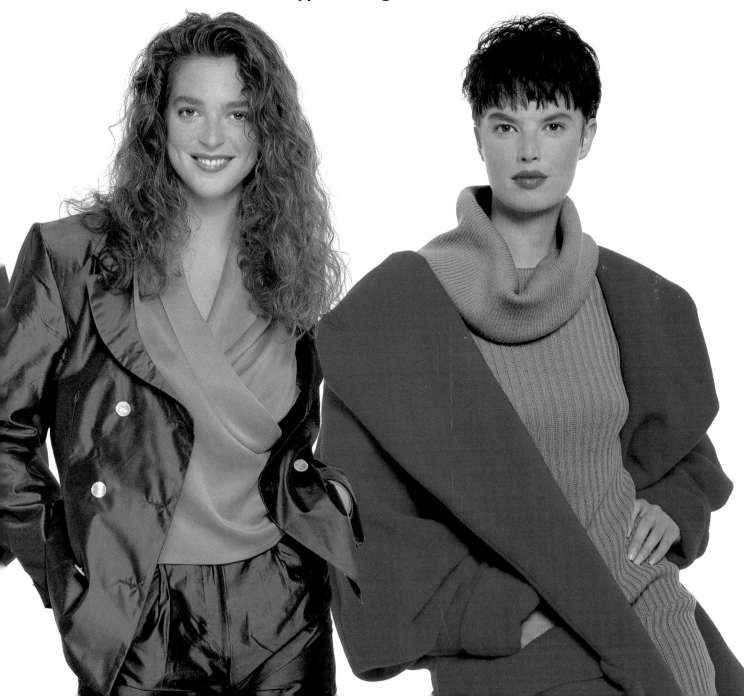

Introduction

Every woman has her favourite colours. The tricky thing is that the colours to which we may feel drawn may not necessarily be the same as those which suit us, flatter us and make us look beautiful. Indeed there are colours that not only suit us but in which we look exceptional! This book is designed to help you discover your own, ideal colour type – divided into the 'seasons' Spring, Summer, Autumn and Winter – whether 'cold' or 'warm' colours suit you best and in which colours you, too, can look exceptional. In 'The Colours of Clothes' you will find practical hints and suggestions for buying clothes – it is particularly annoying and expensive to choose the 'wrong' colour – and there are many recommendations about colours for a basic wardrobe for each type, as well as suggestions for the most attractive colour combinations. The tips in the chapter 'Cosmetic Colours' are stylish and classical and you may prefer one colour option over others, but remember – at all times your own 'season' colour palette remains the same. These suggestions also apply for jewellery and for glasses. And if you are considering having your hair highlighted or tinted, read which colours will suit you best. You may be surprised! Finally, at the end of the book you will find eight pull-out coloured cards which will help you discover your own colour 'season' and which are intended to help you when shopping for clothes. Have fun!

Contents

THE FOUR COLOUR TYPES

Every person is distinctive. Everyone looks different; everyone has their own colouring. Despite this we can all be classified into one of four different types or 'seasons', each of which has a particular relationship to colours. Colours that suit you better than others.

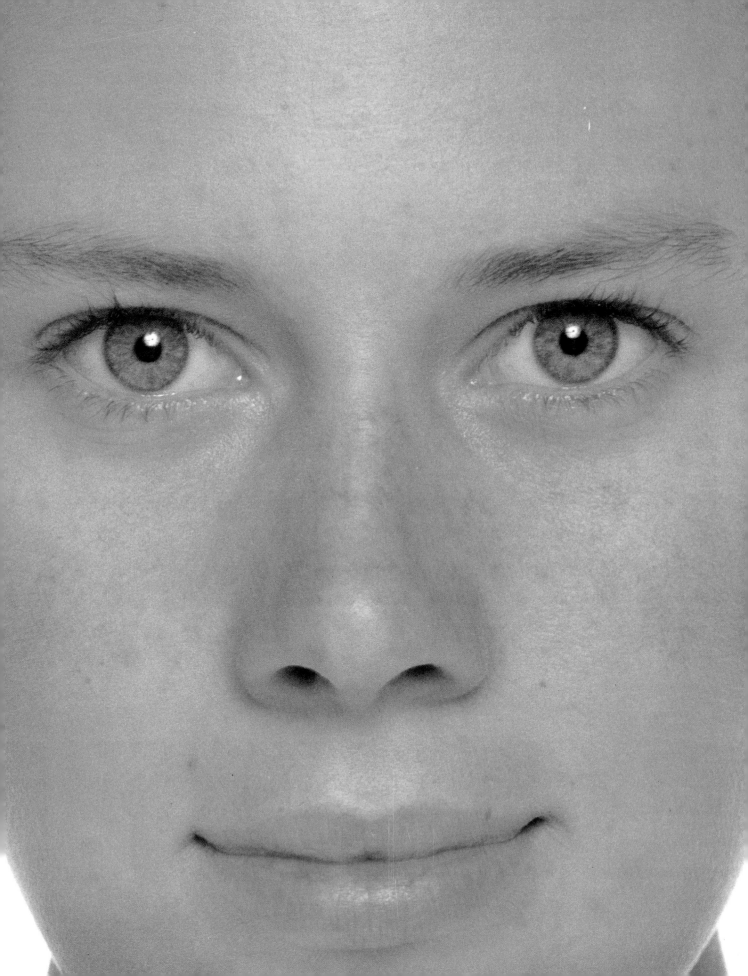

The harmony of colours

From the first to the last day of our lives we are surrounded by colours. The rooms in which we live and work, the scene outside our window, the car or the bus we use, the food on our plates and the cat on our lap, the books on the shelf and the flowers on the table – all these colours overwhelm us daily. Usually we do not take any notice of the individual colours, except when we find the combination of colours especially attractive, or if they particularly disturb us.

The feeling for suitable colour combinations seems to be something with which we are born. Without even thinking about it, we find a particular colour combination harmonious, but another may offend us ... or our soul. Perhaps the reason for this is that nature has always provided us with magnificent examples of colour combinations. Surely no-one would dream of saying, when gazing at a gentle grey-blue veiled mountain scene, 'But that tree in the foreground, with its bright red autumn leaves, is totally out of place'.

No-one finds the illuminating colours of a sunset with all its many shades from brilliant red through yellow to a soft and gentle mauve to be gaudy or jarring. Indeed, it never occurs to us that a meadow full of poppies could be considered 'loud'.

Every colour combination in nature, whether loud or gentle, is harmonious.

But it is quite different when we consider colours we have mixed ourselves. Sometimes we know something is not quite right, that the colours are not harmonious. Indeed, and without our realising it, they may even make us feel aggressive or make someone appear inconspicuous and disagreeable. We will not concern ourselves in this book with architecture or interior design (though there is a lot to be said on both), but only with the colours that we – by choice – wear as well as the natural colours of our skin, hair and eyes.

Have you ever given any thought to the fact that you, too, give an impression through your individual choice of colours? For example, we all have our own particular skin tone which is determined by a number of factors including melanin (the colouring of skin cells). When the sun shines these melanin cells develop as a protection against the sun, causing our tans.

Another factor is haemoglobin, the red 'colouring' in blood, which can sometimes be seen through very pale skin. It doesn't matter whether you have just tanned or are winter pale, the basic colour tone of your skin always remains the same: tinges of the complexion will be either cool and bluish (and in the sun rather ashen) or warm and golden. (To find out how you can determine your own skin colour, read from page 12.)

The natural colours of the skin, hair and eyes are all found on the same scale.

Each human being is a natural piece of 'art' – skin, hair and eye colour derive from the same colour scale. Everything is harmoniously combined: it is we who disturb this harmony. Check what happens when you wear a blue-red lipstick with a sallow face, or an orange blouse with a cool complexion. You look sickly.

Why do we sometimes make such mistakes, when we actually have an inbred sense for the harmony of colours? Why does our eye for colour so often let us down?

There are a number of different reasons. Certainly, it is difficult to be objective about ourselves. Even if we look a thousand times into the mirror, with clothes or without, in jeans, in a dress or in a bikini, with a terrific make-up or none, with a holiday face or after a sleepless night, we still may not really know how we look to others. It is as though our image in the mirror is layered over with other, inner pictures: how we would like to look, an exaggerated self-criticism, whether we could look like the latest model of the day ...

Another reason why we may dress incorrectly is because unconsciously we choose colours that may not suit us. We may feel almost magically drawn to a bright, clear green, but it could make us look very pale – it is a terrific colour in itself but 'kills' the colour tones in our hair, skin and eyes. And someone else may prefer the warm, cosy aura of dark, earthy colours and may not believe that a cool, pastel blue could suit them far better.

Many children love red; later on they prefer blue. Older people, on the other hand, like pastel colours. It seems 'natural'.

Our taste in colours may often change throughout our lives. Perhaps you remember that nearly all children love the bright primaries – red and yellow. When they reach puberty they are drawn by the melancholy effects of blue. During adulthood their favourite colours may change many times and then when older, many turn to pastel colours. Our 'inner' colours change, but the basic tone of our skin remains the same all our life.

And even when our own hair turns grey, we have our own individual grey hues that complement our skin and eye colours. Natural – at all stages of our lives.

Naturally, we use our clothes to express our moods – to enhance them or change them in some way. Perhaps we choose a bright yellow blouse believing this jolly colour will cheer us up or will at least have the effect of making those around us think that everything is going well. Or there may be a certain colour that we cannot bear when we are feeling low: the mood is grey, the clothes as well, and we don't care whether red looks better or not. But even when, after reading this book, you discover which colours suit you and which do not, don't see this as a rigid set of rules. There will be days when you will want to ignore it all and, if it makes you feel better, do so!

The same can be said for women who love to wear black. Pure black actually suits only about a quarter of all women; for others it can appear tiring and ageing. But black is more than a fashion colour, it is a mark of distinction. Black can mark you out from the colourful masses; it means being different, and sometimes we need to stand out. There are various ways of livening up black – with the use of colourful shawls or other accessories – but we are talking about colour. Perhaps, just for once, lovers of black might consider trying the colour 'season' which really suits their appearance. They may be surprised.

Naturally, how we view fashion trends also influences the way we choose colours. Twice a year particular colours will be promoted by magazines and designers. If aubergine, neon pink, or emerald green happen to be in fashion, then these colours will be seen everywhere for at least one season: in every shop window and in every restaurant, on bags and in skirts, in ribbons, sweaters and bathing costumes. Don't be brain-washed.

In some colours we look good; in others, fantastic. Whether these are fashionable colours or not is irrelevant.

In time, the eye becomes accustomed to colours and while it is obvious that aubergine, neon pink or emerald green do not suit everyone, many women will buy something in these 'fashionable' colours. They are simply not able to resist joining in the trend. They know no-one will notice they haven't got a coat in aubergine but perhaps someone will say, 'You look terrific in your blue coat.' But aubergine is the fashionable colour, not blue.

There are many colours that suit you, but some are better for you than others. This is also true for cosmetics as well as clothes. Why should you be content with something good, when for the same price you can have something better?

Take your time to look at the four women on the opposite page. In one photograph they are wearing clothes and make-up that do not suit them; in the other, the clothes and make-up flatter and complement them. Quite honestly, none of them looks ugly in any of the photos – a beautiful person cannot be easily changed for the worse. Nevertheless, there is a very clear difference: in colours suitable for their colour type they simply look a lot more attractive and are generally more harmonious. They have more radiance. There is a feeling that everything is just right, that these colours suit this person. And this is what this book is all about.

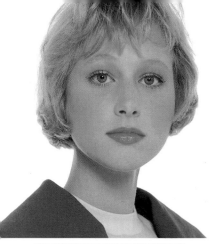
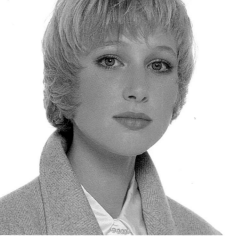

The styling in the left hand photograph is good, but the hard colour contrast does not flatter a naturally delicate appearance – this is achieved by the softer colours in the picture on the right.

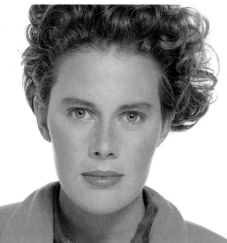
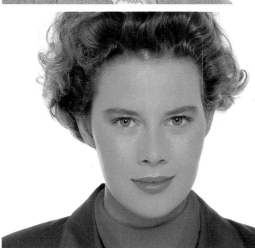

A lot of brown powder and rouge on a natural, strongly toned skin (photo left) certainly looks more sporty, but also a little crude. Finer and more suited to her type is the cooler make-up on the right.

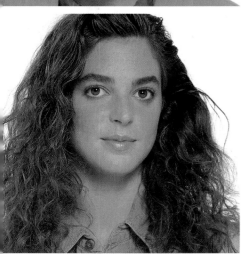
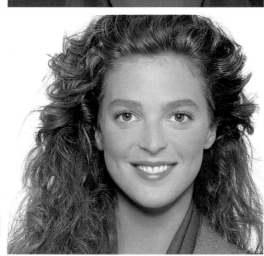

Anyone with reddish hair tends to over- or under-emphasise and sometimes chooses colours for either an inconspicuous, natural appeal or chooses extreme effects such as lilac mother-of-pearl (photo left). Deep, rich colours, such as those on the right, give this person a great deal more contour.

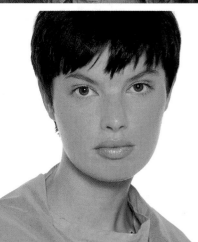
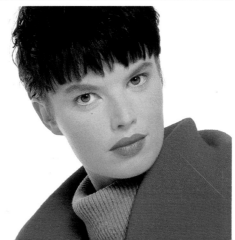

A woman with intensive natural colours – dark hair and eyes, light complexion – should emphasise these contrasts. In the subdued colours on the left the effect is boring; on the right, much more exciting.

The colours of the seasons

The idea of colour counselling comes from America, as does the suggestion to name the individual colour types after the four seasons – Spring, Summer, Autumn, and Winter. They could just as easily be distinguished as type 1, type 2, type 3 and type 4 or A, B, C, and D, but the 'season' theme has a particular appeal and is popular with many people. The idea is that one particular season suits each one of us particularly well: the intensive, contrast-rich and cool tones of winter; or the more subdued, vapoury colours of summer; the warm clarity of spring or the shining, yet earthy colours of autumn.

The most important, but also the most difficult decision – do warm or cold colours suit me best?

Incidentally, this will have nothing to do with when you were born or which is your favourite season. It is instead a quite arbitrary classification, but one which is relevant and very personal. It rests principally on two conditions: the colour of your complexion and the intensity and depth of that colour. If your skin has a yellow, almost golden undertone, then warm colours will harmonise well with your colouring, whilst alongside cool colours your skin will lose its gentle golden tone and appear sallow. If your skin has a bluish tinge to it and an almost invisible grey tone, then cool colours will suit you; however, your skin will appear pale alongside warm shades.

The nuances of the cooler colour palette suit the Winter and Summer type best. Spring and Autumn women on the other hand look better in warm colours.

And what about skin intensity and depth of colour? Imagine for a moment the colour yellow. What do you see? There is the radiant, strong, yolk yellow; the cooler lemon yellow; creamy yellow of vanilla ice-cream; icy light yellow, warm slightly red maize yellow; golden yellow, and mustard yellow ... You can see the difference between a strong yellow tone, such as yolk yellow which 'shouts' at you, and a rather reserved, very gentle yellow such as vanilla.

Some women look magnificent in starkly contrasting colours, but others may 'disappear' behind them. The dress, its colour and its pattern are seen, but not the person. Such people need powdery, softer tones and quiet patterns – then we see the whole person and not just the dress.

Every colour scale has its own mood. Its colours have a soft or a strong effect, flowery or earthy.

In the case of the Summer and Winter colour types for whom cool tones are best suited, Winter is best in strong contrasts – think of bare, dark branches bearing frosty red fruit against the white of the snow.

The Summer type can also use cool tones, but with more subdued, softer, pastel colours – like a damp mist stretched out across the fields by the sun.

For Spring and Autumn types for whom warmer tones are best, Autumn prefers the more powerful colours – it represents the not-too-heavy brightness of autumn leaves lying on the brown earth.

EVERYWHERE COLOURS, COLOURS...13

To the Spring types belong the clear, gentle tones, a subtle clarity of light – the true colours of spring flowers.

To decide your colour type is simple. At the end of this book you will find a colour chart with the four colour palettes on the front and the reverse sides. Cut it in half along its length.

Place the colour scales next to each other, turn them around and combine them to suit yourself – do you see a difference between the cooler and the warmer shades, powdery and clear colours and between soft and strong colours? Every strip of colour produces its own characteristic mood. It could be that you find one or the other series of colours attractive, but reject a third.

Perhaps you have chosen the correct colours instinctively. But this is not necessarily so – do not decide yet. The final decision must be made when you know more about your type.

And another thing may occur to you. The colours are subdivided into seasonal palettes, so on every palette there is (with few exceptions) every colour. This means whichever type you are, you can wear any colour – it depends only on the shade of that colour.

Everywhere colours, colours…

When you first begin to notice colours you will notice something interesting - suddenly you will be aware of every colour and colour combination you see and which previously you would have ignored.

You will be in a restaurant and begin to wonder why the man at the next table particularly chose to wear a grass-green shirt, why the colours of the curtains clash so strongly with that of the floor and why the woman in the corner has had her hair bleached, although she has such a red face. When you are watching the news you may wonder why the mauve sweater worn by the announcer yesterday didn't suit her as well as the pink blouse she is wearing today? Which colour type is she? (Don't forget that it is very difficult to assess colour from the television screen as the lighting and make-up play a large role.)

Maybe your husband and friends find it annoying if you continually criticise other people's colours. If so - ignore them! This initial reaction will go away. And it is necessary to be this critical. You will become increasingly involved with colours, the effects of colours, how colours look alongside each other, how the effect is increased or decreased when specific colours are coordinated and how much more alive and full of expression colours can make you. Keep your eyes open; you will become more aware and sensitive and your sense of colour will grow day by day.

This is what the Spring type looks like

The Spring woman has something delicate and fragile about her – whatever her size or weight. It is her skin which gives this impression: it is light, almost pale and transparent, has no blue in it but always a yellow to gentle golden undertone. Some Spring types have an almost ivory complexion, others may have tinges of red. The romantic comparison with a peach is not out of place: many women of this type have a rosy peach-coloured blush over the cheeks (but remember – the red of the cheeks never has a bluish pink tone).

Many Spring women also suffer from red blotches on their skin when excited. Others will have freckles which, if looked at closely, are not grey-brown, but golden brown. Despite this sensitive tender skin, women of this type often tan very quickly.

Most Spring types have blonde hair: flaxen, straw blonde, golden blond, beige-blonde, or strawberry blonde – the nuances vary.

What other women pay good money for, the Spring woman will often be born with – light golden strands in the hair or golden yellow tips bleached by the sun. Even as their hair ages it never becomes mousey; it always keeps its golden tinge. What is the colour of the eyes of the Spring type? As the palette is large – from blue or blue-turquoise and grey-green to golden brown – any colour is possible (very occasionally the eyes are a quite dark and stunning intense green).

Photo right:
The Spring woman without make up has a delicate, almost transparent complexion but often with a tinge of a clear peach-coloured cheek blush. The hair always retains a golden shimmer even if it darkens with age.

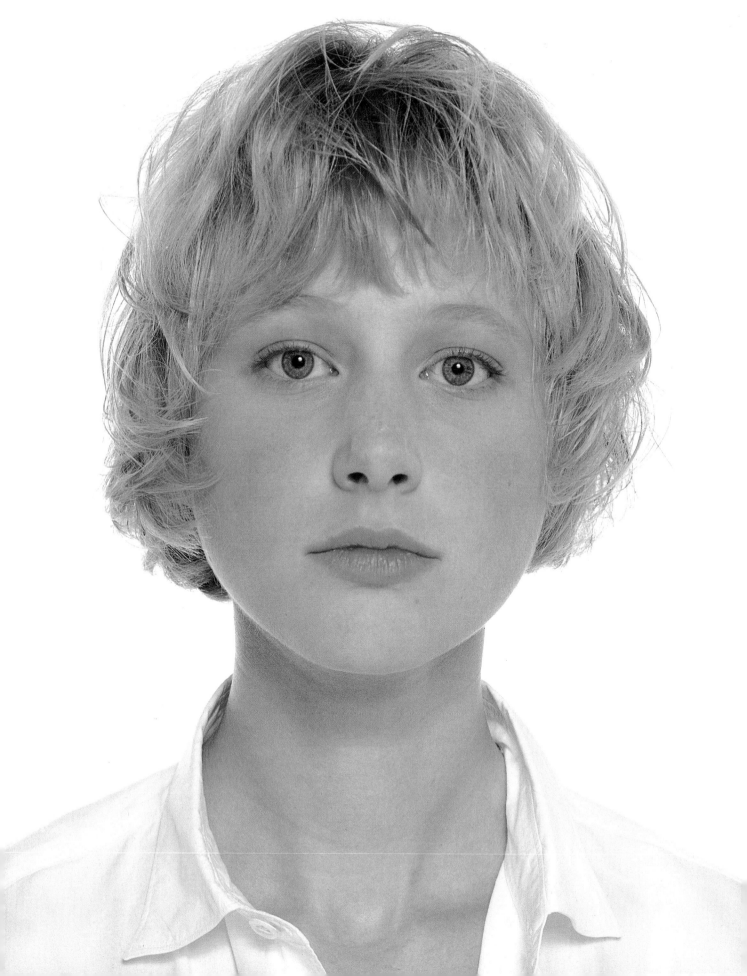

This is what the Summer type looks like

Women classified as a Summer type are frequently found in northern Europe. They may have very different characteristics but common to all is a bluish undertone to the skin and a somewhat ashy instead of golden shine to the hair. There are Summer types with a delicately light, almost milk-white complexion; others by contrast have a rosy skin. Summer women with an olive tint to the skin will have difficulty deciding their type; they quickly become a gentle brown in the sun so tend to believe they have a yellow skin undertone. Freckles are likely to be grey-brown, never golden brown like the Spring types! Except for the pale, white-skinned Summer type, all Summer types tan easily, with their skin adopting a hazelnut tone (the brown of the Spring type, on the other hand, is somewhat reddish!) Many Summer types are disappointed with the colour of their hair and tend to experiment with different tones – they may believe their hair is mousey. If Summer types were blonde as children, then it will have been platinum blonde without even a tinge of yellow. Very few retain this blonde hair; with most Summer types the hair changes and becomes much darker – ash blonde or middle to dark brown. Don't be confused if in the sun you discover reddish highlights in your hair! These are red pigments which, in the case of middle Europeans, usually shows up in the sunshine – the black hair of Asians picks up a blue shimmer. The eye colour of the Summer type? Often grey-blue, light blue, grey-petrol, blue-green, but also hazelnut brown. A characteristic of the Summer type is that their eyes appear lightly overcast; the whites of the eyes tend to be rather milky and do not stand in sharp contrast to the iris.

Photo right: The Summer type without make-up. Generally, the complexion is more strongly pigmented than the Spring type. If the skin has freckles, these tend to be grey rather than golden. Typically, the hair colour will be ash blonde or ash brown, both with cool effect.

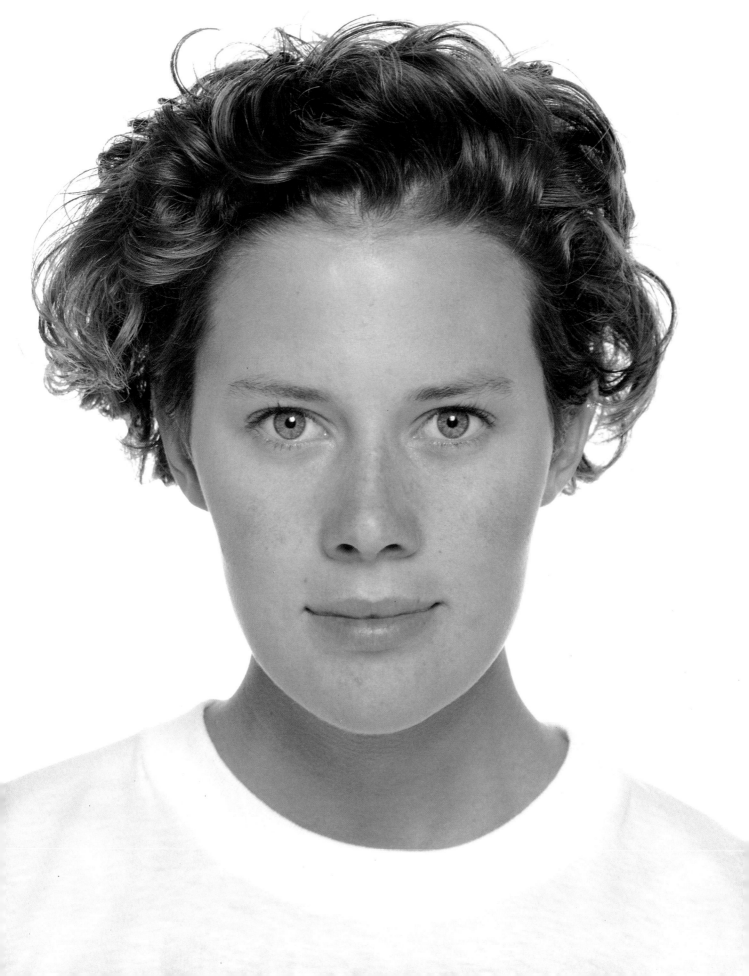

This is what the Autumn type looks like

Among the four types, the Autumn type is the attractive 'chameleon' for, depending upon her style, she can make changes like no other type. Some Autumn women, depending on the intensity of hair and eye colours, look extremely attractive without make-up; others at first glance may not stand out but with just a touch of colour they quickly begin to look very attractive indeed. All Autumn types will have a golden-yellow, warm undertone to the skin; the complexion appears to be pale and transparent (sometimes with gentle reddish freckles) or tends towards a tender champagne tone. Many other women of this type have a more intensive skin colour – a powerful golden beige or peach, similar to some Spring types, but more pronounced. There is, however, another difference: the skin of the Spring type tends to have a rosy overtone to it, often with peach-coloured cheeks; Autumn types rarely have a natural red colour in the cheeks.

And where Spring skin types quickly tan, usually Autumn types will just as quickly get sunburnt.

The characteristic hair colour for this type is red – from carrot red through copper red to chestnut brown. Naturally, there are also women of this type who have middle to dark brown hair, but they always retain reddish golden highlights! Their complexions, too, will have this warm tinge in contrast to the cooler effect of Summer's skin type with their silver-ashy hair tints.

The eye colours of the Autumn type? In many cases the eyes are particularly impressive – they are always very intense, sometimes glass-clear, sometimes glowing. The colour palette stretches from shining light blue, steel blue and petrol through amber to a light slate-green and full olive, from golden brown to an intense dark brown. Typical for many Autumn types is also a blotched iris with golden streaks.

Photo right: The Autumn type without make-up. Red or honey coloured hair, intensive eyes in a warm colour, pale yellow or brownish skin are common characteristics. When the Autumn type has freckles, which is often the case, they are always golden brown.

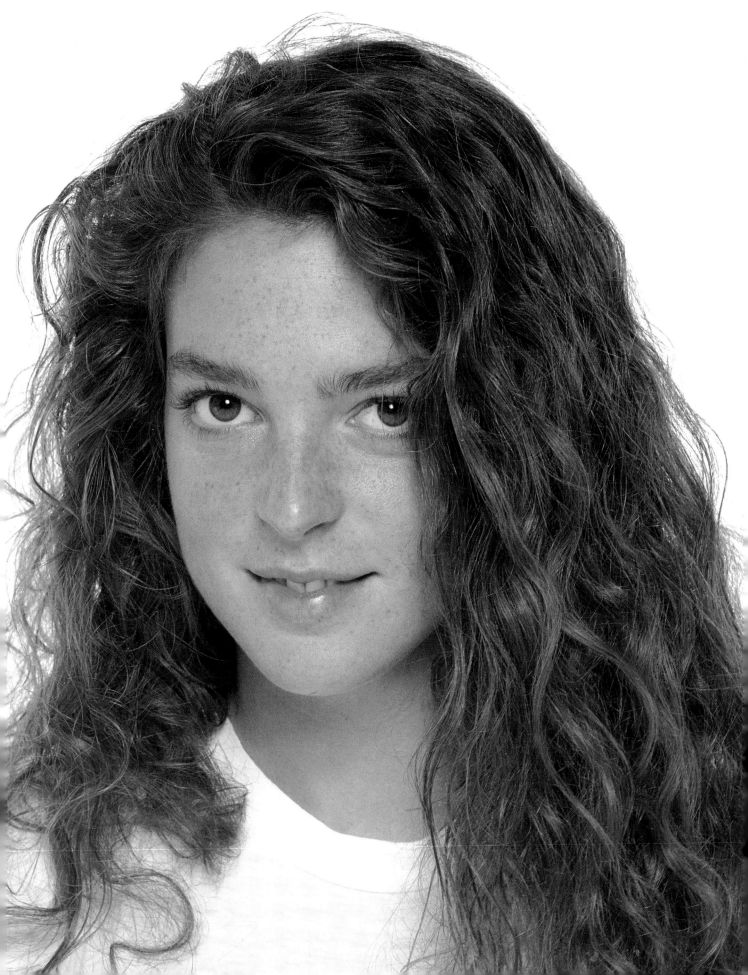

This is what the Winter type looks like

'White as snow and black as charcoal' – Snow White had the typical characteristics of the Winter type. These women are fascinating because of their strong dramatic contrasts: light skin, dark hair and intense iris colours with clear whites to their eyes. The undertone of the skin is always a cool blue. It is sometimes difficult to see this clearly – with their white skin the Winter type never tans well; instead they often turn a soft brown shade which can disguise the bluish undertone in their skin.

Sometimes this blueness to the skin only becomes clear when comparing it with the warm golden shimmer in the skin of the Spring type. Whether or not their skin is pale or olive-tinged Winter's skin will always look transparent and cool – like porcelain. Only barely does it show a wisp of blush on the cheeks. Most Winter women like dark hair: blue-black, deep black, black-brown and dark brown, and while some may have been very blonde as children the hair becomes darker with age until reaching a middle brown. The Winter woman will always have a cool ashy hair tone even if in strong sunlight a red shimmer appears. These red tones, which can also appear in strongly worn hair ends, come from the deep-lying pigments of the hair and actually have little to do with the actual colour of the hair.

The eye colour of the Winter type? Always clear, intense and distinct. The most common eye colours are ice blue, violet blue, deep blue, unmixed grey, glass-clear green and naturally dark and black-brown. Mixed colours, for example grey-green, are rare, but even these are never as creamy and subdued as the Summer type, always maintaining a strong contrast to the clear white of the eye.

Photo right: The Winter type without make-up. Even a gently tanned complexion is cool and light like porcelain, never warm and golden. However, the most important characteristics are the contrasts – dark hair with a light skin, strong iris colour with clear eye white.

Spring colour range

nd use them as instructed to find your colour type.

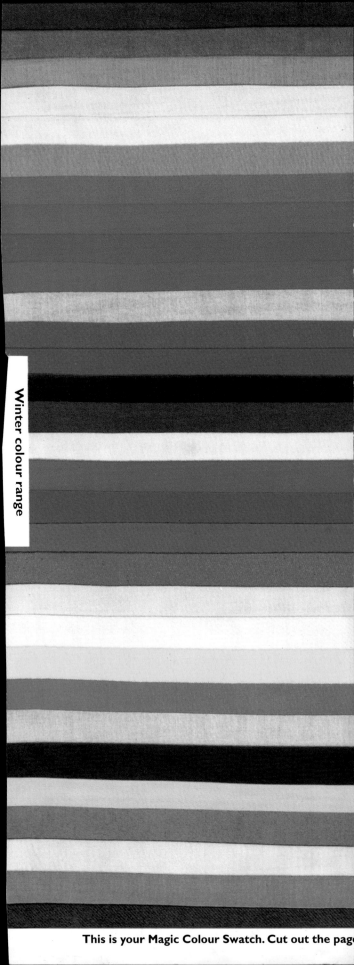

Winter colour range

This is your Magic Colour Swatch. Cut out the page

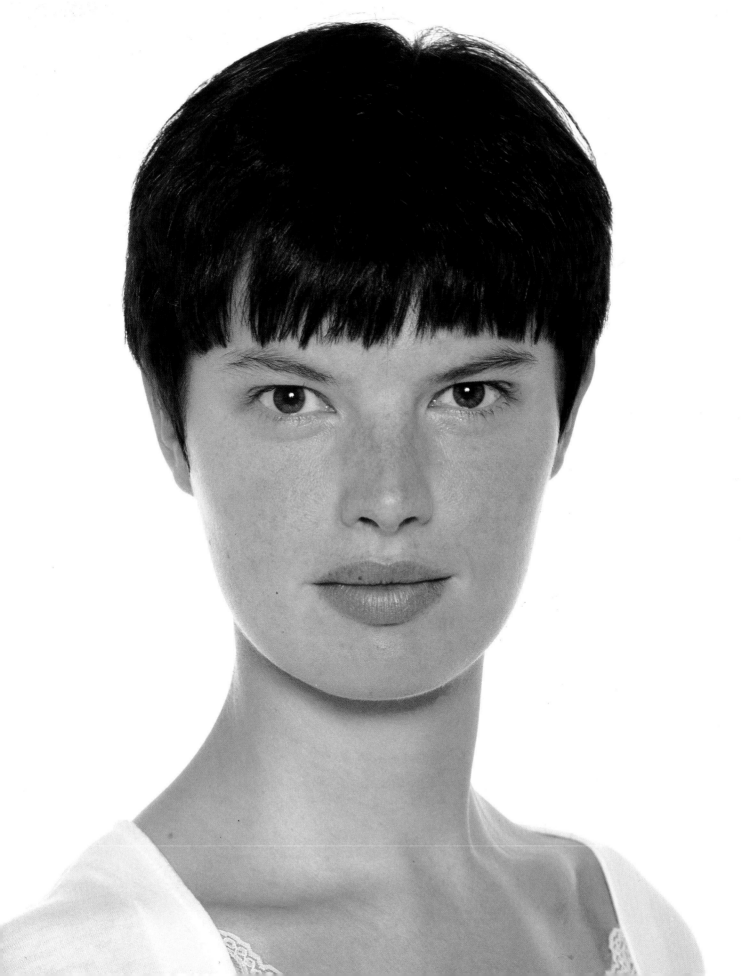

FIND THE RIGHT COLOUR TYPE

Generally speaking every woman can wear any colour she likes. It simply depends which shade of colour she chooses. But there are a few rules that should be taken into account when selecting the right colour for you, and in order to understand the characteristics within colour groups, it is necessary to learn to see them in a quite new way.

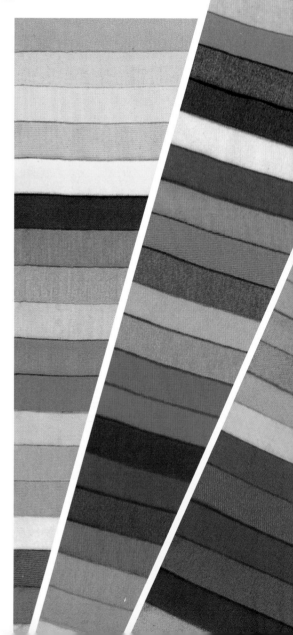

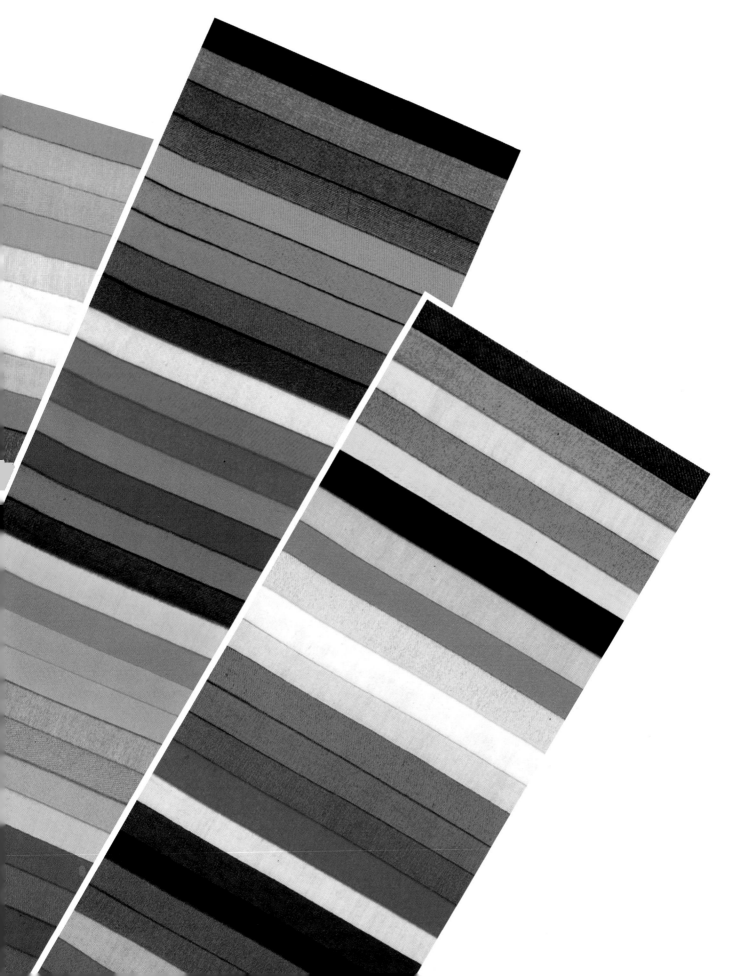

What colour type am I?

Perhaps you have already recognised yourself from the preceding description of the four 'season' types. Or you may be wondering whether your hair really does have golden highlights? Or if your skin is yellow or just tanned? And where is the blue tinge you should recognise? To help you the following section is divided into two parts – first, how to see colours as they really are and second, which colours suit you.

The description of how to learn to look at colours is very important. From the moment we wake until we go to bed we are saturated with colour without really being conscious of all the various nuances of those colours.

Have you taken out the colour charts at the end of the book? Now take the chart with the four different coloured strips (for the four 'season' types on the front and back) which you have cut lengthways down the middle.

Look at them. Turn them around. Compare and combine them in several different ways.

Pink or bluish rose is a pronounced cool colour. It clashes with all warm tones.

Lay these coloured strips open as you continue to read, and play around with them.

Automatically you will find yourself developing a feeling for the individual colour groups. Are you able to recognise that two colour groups harmonise with each other and that two others clash? There are two colour scales with warm colours for the seasons Spring and Autumn and two scales with cool colours for Summer and Winter. Putting warm colours next to each other is harmonious; the same goes for cold colours. A combination of Winter (cold colours)

Salmon rose or apricot is the warmest rose tone. It has a strong yellow tint; not 'cold' like the bluish-pink opposite.

correct colour tone has been chosen. The same goes for blue, green, yellow and all other colours – in each colour there are warm shades and cool shades. The point to remember is to select the right colour shade for your type.

Something else will strike you about the coloured strips: their effect differs – one is gentle, the other more intense. The examples classified as Summer and Winter are both cool colour ranges but are vastly different in depth. The scale of the Summer range contains subdued, almost smokey tones; those of Winter are clear and pure. Those colours on the Spring and Autumn scale are warm: the Spring colours are delicate and fresh, with Autumn colours earthy and full.

Now take the other seven colour charts – on the front and reverse sides there are four red tones, four blue tones, four green tones, a rose and an apricot. Can you see the differences? On one side each chart has a warm colour tone, on the other a cool one. Also the intensity of the colours is different – some are quite powerful and clear, others are soft and subdued.

and Autumn (warm colours) greatly disturbs our sense of colour.

Place the chart in such a way that the red tones of Winter and Autumn are next to each other. Do you see the differences?

The red of Winter is much more decisive, clearer and above all bluer. It tends towards a cyclamen red. Now add to this a cool pink and an icy rose.

Compare this with the red of Autumn. It is far softer and warmer! The most powerful reds – do you see the brown to yellow tones in them? – do not become more blue alongside the lighter shades but instead appear orange, apricot and salmon. No question about it – both Winter and Autumn types can wear red. It suits them both particularly well but only if the

Each of the single colour tones harmonises with a seasonal scale. Try it out! Open pages 28–29: here you will find all four colour scales printed next to each other. Place each one of the charts in the place drawn in for them, or mix them around as you wish. Can you see the effect? All the warm colours harmonise with the colour scales of the seasons Spring and Autumn; all the cold ones with the cooler colour scales of Summer and Winter. For example, an Autumn green (warm) clashes with the Summer colours (cold). You will quickly recognise harmony and disharmony using the apricot colour scales. Warm apricot harmonises with the Spring and Autumn colours, whereas against the Summer and Winter it has a quite jarring effect. Try it for yourself; learn to assess your colours.

Are you now prepared for a test?

In order to find out which of the four season types you are, you must prepare yourself properly and do a colour test. But it is best to read through the chapter first before you start.

First, your position; ideally you should sit in front of a large mirror at a north-facing window as colours cannot be properly assessed in bright sunlight (artists' studios always face north for this very reason).

Please only do this test during the day, as artificial light falsifies the colours. Naturally, you should remove all make-up.

Have you any skin blemishes or red veins? Do not cover these up; you will only be able to truly discover your colour type if you appear as you really are. Next, your hair – if natural you will find the test easy. However, dyed, coloured or bleached hair can falsify the test result. Some colour counsellors cover the hair with a scarf in a neutral colour at this point: we advise against this as we believe the colour of the scarf may unconsciously influence the test.

Comb your hair straight off your face. Can you see a natural growing hair line? So much the better! Do the test wearing just a blouse, or wrap yourself up – the shoulders must remain free – in a towel, a man's shirt, a hand towel or something similar.

The important thing to remember is that the material must have no colour in it. Any such colour will distract you. The ideal is a clean white with no yellow in it. And before you proceed any further, ask yourself whether you want to do the test on your own or whether you would prefer extra help and judgement?

Sometimes it is fun to do this test with friends – a real 'Colour Counselling party' – where you can assist and advise each other. Obviously this is a lot of fun but it is doubtful whether it makes a lot of sense. Friends will certainly have a more objective judgement but the danger is that they may unconsciously transfer their own favourite colours on to you. And these will not necessarily be the colours that really suit you!

We would advise you to do the test quietly on your own at first. You can always repeat it with friends afterwards if you wish.

The same is true for men wanting to be helpful in this test as there are probably few who can make an objective judgement about their loved ones! For example, your partner may have happy memories of the blue sweater you used to wear when he first knew you. You know it yourself – a colour you feel suits you is not necessarily the best for your type!

Often we believe that a colour suits us well – just because someone told us so.

In colour counselling studios pieces of differently-coloured fabrics are sometimes used, placed on customers' shoulders. As no one will have a complete range of coloured cloths in all the many colour shades, it is necessary to use the colour chart in the self-test in order to see which colours harmonise with your face and which do not. How is this done?

It is fairly easy – sit comfortably in the correct daylight before the mirror, hold one chart after another under the chin and carefully watch what happens to your face. Which chart livens it up? Which makes it look more tired?

If you are wearing the right colours people will notice your face: not your clothes.

Are you having difficulties doing this test? Don't worry: to properly assess yourself is tricky. Take heart and go through the procedure a few times or read the chapter again. It will help.

The important things to remember when doing the test:

● When looking in the mirror, always look at your face and not at the colour chart! This is not at all easy but remember – you are looking for the effect the chart has on your face (not the colour chart itself).

● Try to free yourself from any long-held prejudices about individual colours. The important thing about this test is not which colour you like or dislike, which colours are in your wardrobe or which you feel you would never wear – the one aim of this test is to find out which colour type you are. Don't say, 'I know that colour doesn't suit me'. That is not the point and you need never wear this colour if you don't wish to; you are testing the colour charts to discover your type.

● Please do not give up if you find it hard to see any differences in the charts. Even when working in studio conditions, professional colour counsellors may make several attempts until – together with the customer – they come to a decision. So, please take your time, repeat the test several times if you wish, make your decision and then check it at your leisure. Given time you will develop a feeling for what is right!

It is best to begin with the pink chart. Here you will see most clearly the contrast between a bluish and a yellowish tone.

First place the cool rose side and then the warm apricot side under the face and watch what happens to your face with each one:

Does your complexion become yellower? Or rosier? Greyer? Paler?

Do your eyes radiate more intensely? Or are any eye bags seen more clearly? Do the charts have a freshening effect on your face or do you look older? Do skin blemishes look more pronounced?

Does the face appear to sag or look spongy, or does it acquire flattering contours? Do you have the feeling that the colour swamps your face making you look pale and inconspicuous? Remember – you will not be able to see this all in one go, but you will already have begun to pick up some clues.

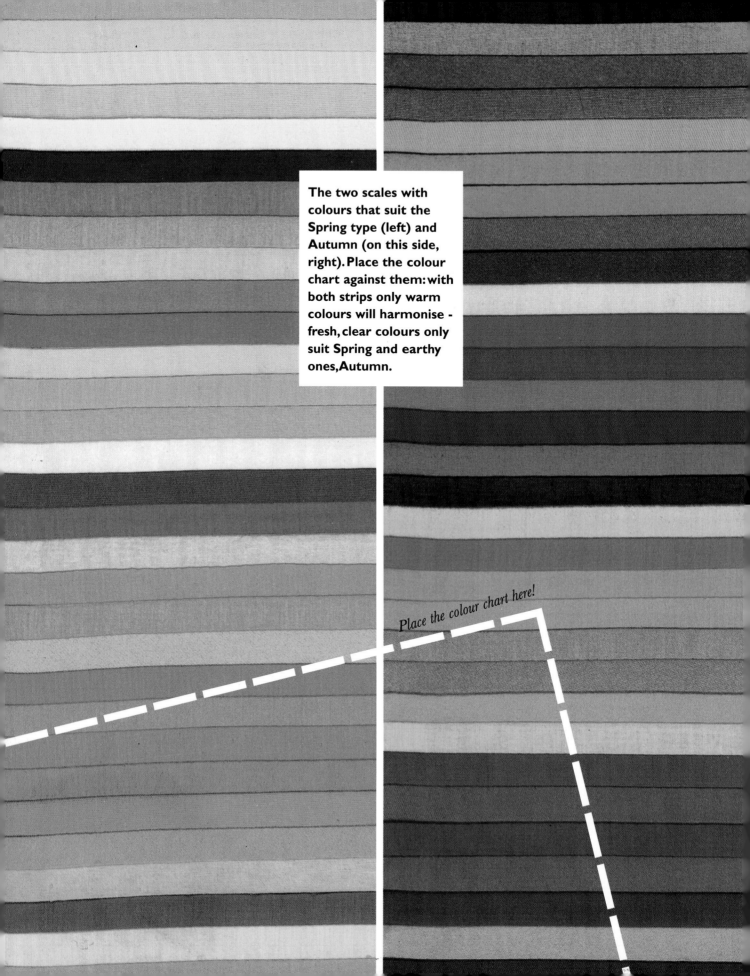

The two scales with colours that suit the **Spring** type (left) and **Autumn** (on this side, right). Place the colour chart against them: with both strips only warm colours will harmonise - fresh, clear colours only suit **Spring** and earthy ones, **Autumn**.

Place the colour chart here!

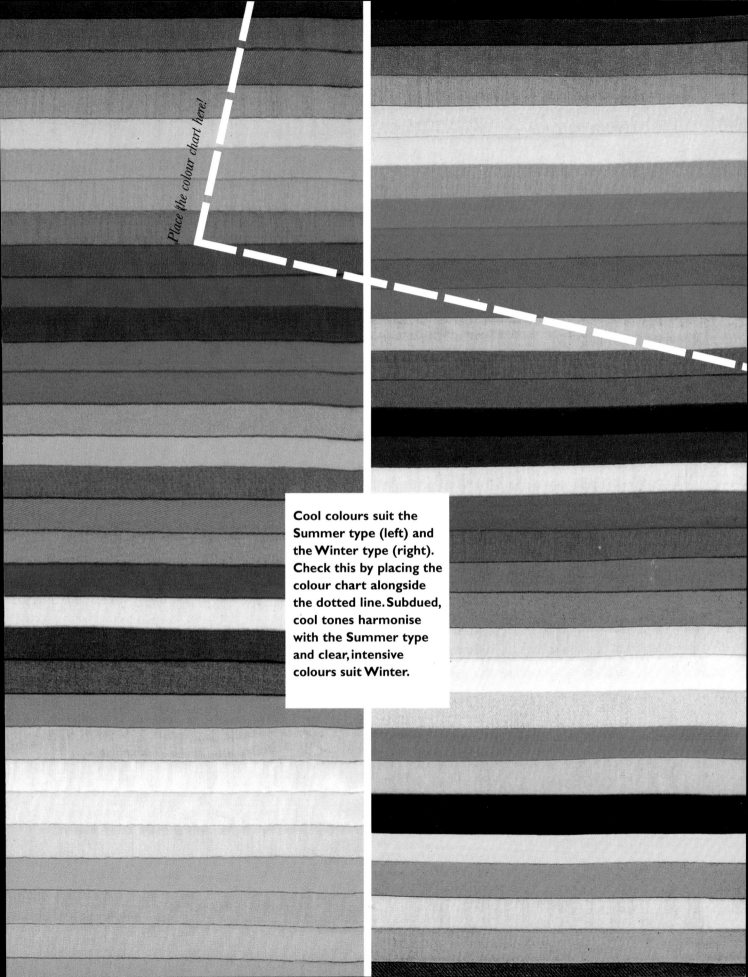

Place the colour chart here!

Cool colours suit the Summer type (left) and the Winter type (right). Check this by placing the colour chart alongside the dotted line. Subdued, cool tones harmonise with the Summer type and clear, intensive colours suit Winter.

Now test the four different tones of red – a colour with the strongest effect. Does a warm red bring life to your face or, by contrast, does a cold red improve you? Perhaps you cannot decide between two red tones. Wait a moment. Take your time and test all the colours on the charts and repeat the whole thing as often as you wish. Each time your 'eye' will improve. The ideal colours for you will suit you so well that when wearing these colours you will be able to go out without wearing any make-up, because it is your face that is seen and not the colour of your dress.

Have you made your choice and decided on a type? Or are you swinging between different seasons? Ask yourself – have I made a mistake? For example, are you remembering a particular coloured dress which is always complimented and which is influencing you now? Be careful...In making your decision you may say, 'But this colour also suits me!' Do not compromise. The important thing is the colours that suit you best; not those which just suit you well! Make notes.

For example, red – spring, blue – summer, green – spring, rose – cool. In this case you would be clearly blonde but still undecided whether you are a Spring or Summer type. That you have chosen a cool rose, speaks more of Summer. Do the test once more and carefully read the descriptions of the individual types. Which really applies to you?

Sometimes it is only possible to determine your skin tone by comparison with other parts of your body.

It is vital to assess the correct skin undertone – a bluish or a yellow-gold tinge. Look at the underside of your arms, at the forehead under a fringe, at your breasts or your stomach!

Colours may only be truly decided when placed alongside comparisons. If this is true in your case, try it. Is your face skin colour cooler or warmer when checked with your arms or stomach? With time you will find this easier to do.

You can check whether you have made a right or wrong season type decision on p.32–39.

If you want to discover which colour suits you best and which should be avoided, you must develop your colour 'eye'! Green is not just green and blue is not just blue. There are hundreds of different shades. On this page you will find just four nuances of each colour. All are identical to the colour tones on the charts at the end of the book, and they harmonise appropriately with the colours of Spring, Summer, Autumn and Winter.

What is important if you want to develop a sense of colour is to recognise if a colour is clear or if it has been toned with another basic colour. And if so, with which? With a warm colour tone (yellow or red) or with a cool one (blue)? Remember: those colours on the two left areas of each coloured square are toned with warm colours; those found on the right with cold ones.

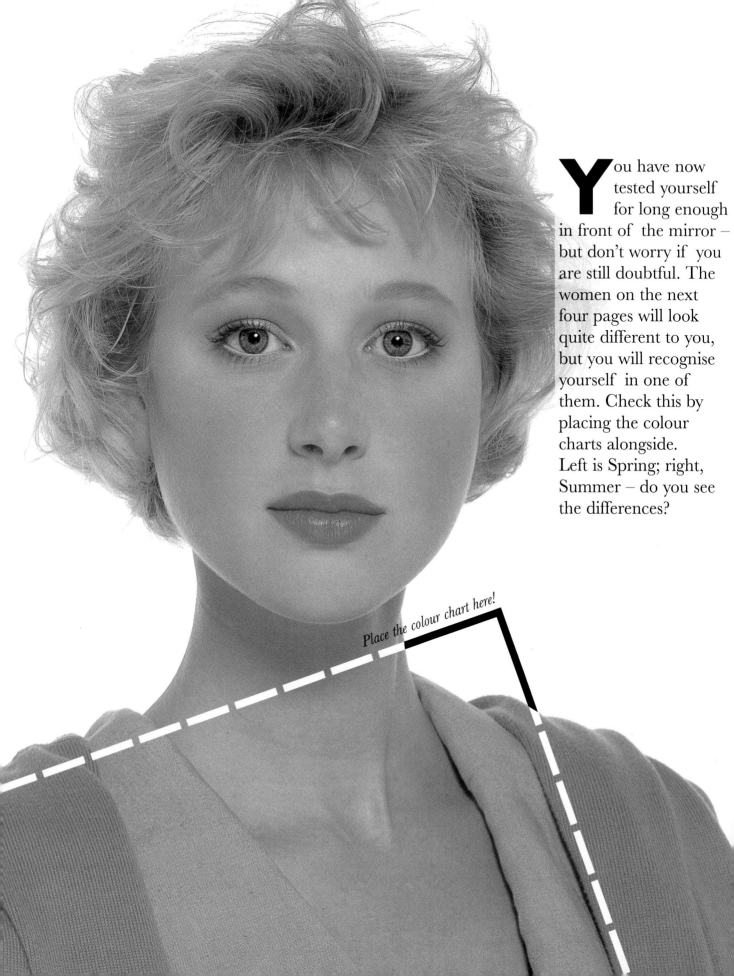

You have now tested yourself for long enough in front of the mirror – but don't worry if you are still doubtful. The women on the next four pages will look quite different to you, but you will recognise yourself in one of them. Check this by placing the colour charts alongside. Left is Spring; right, Summer – do you see the differences?

Place the colour chart here!

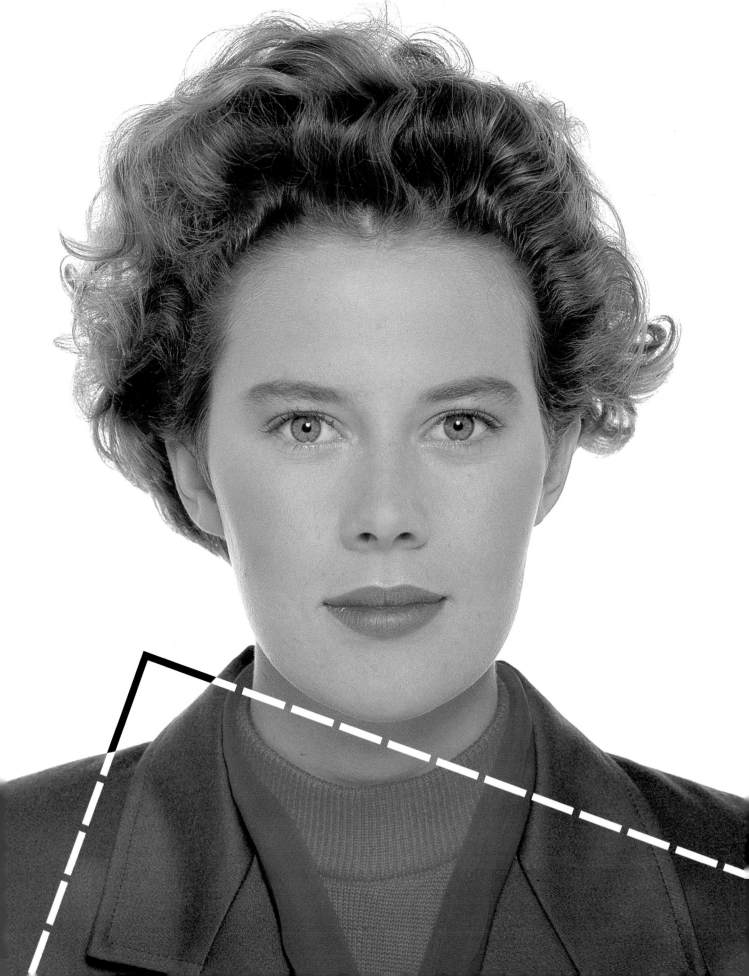

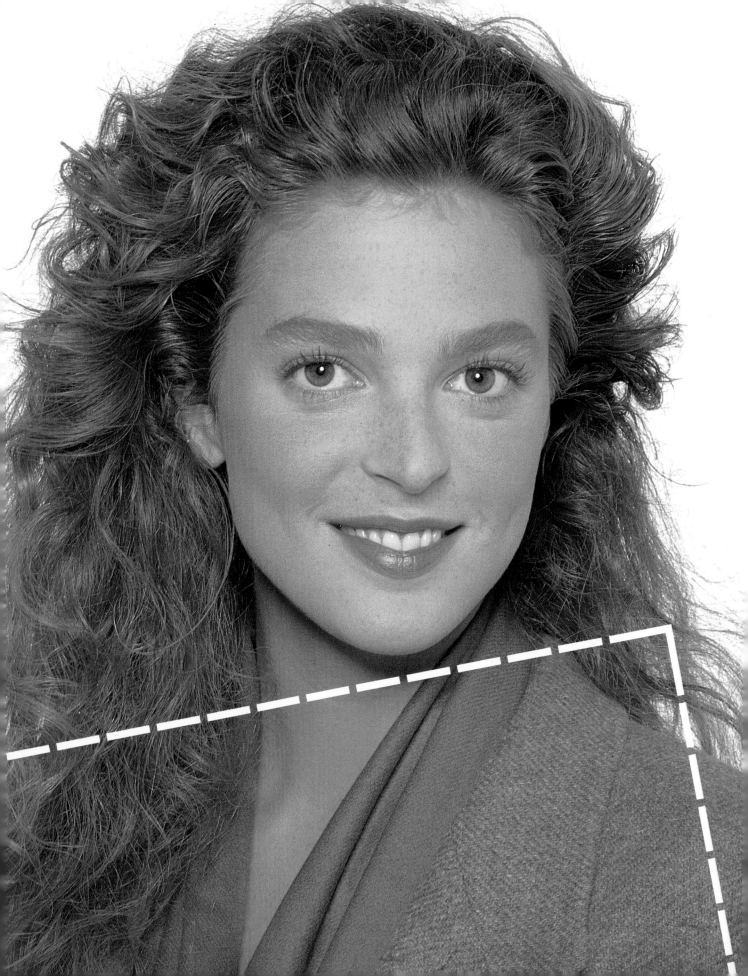

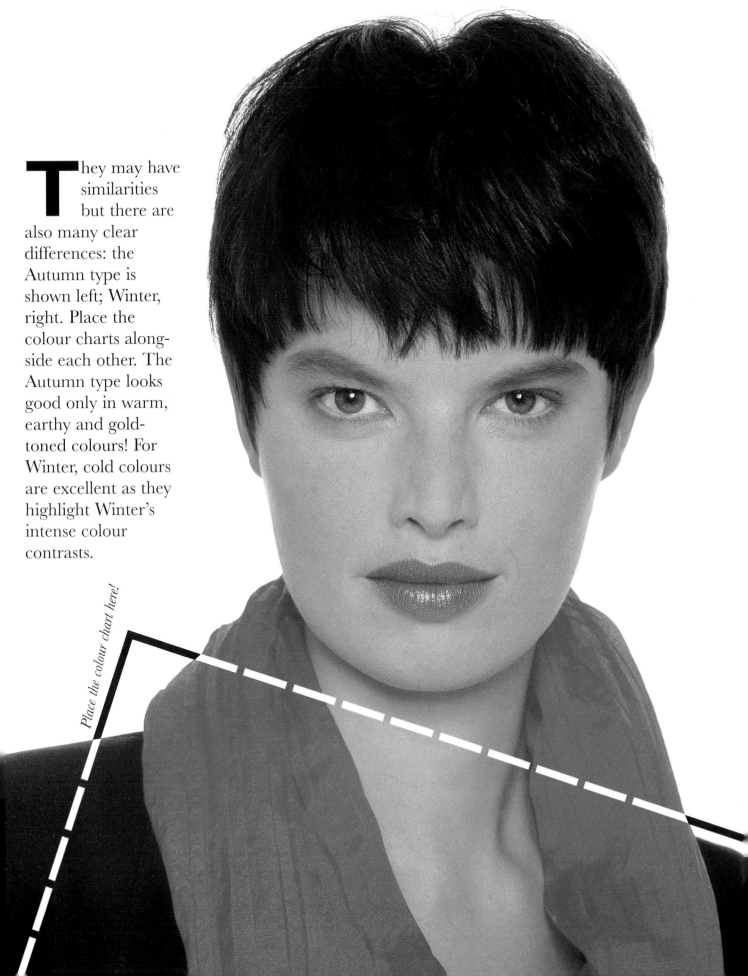

They may have similarities but there are also many clear differences: the Autumn type is shown left; Winter, right. Place the colour charts alongside each other. The Autumn type looks good only in warm, earthy and gold-toned colours! For Winter, cold colours are excellent as they highlight Winter's intense colour contrasts.

Place the colour chart here!

Check again whether your decision is the right one

You have read the descriptions of the four different season types; you have studied the different colour scales of the seasons and have probably discovered which one suits you best. You have tested yourself in front of a mirror with the help of the colour chart (probably several times, on your own or later with a friend) and you have seen the effect of the different red, blue or green tones on the photographs on the preceding pages. Possibly you are now quite certain which colour type you are?

However, there may still be some readers who are unclear. Maybe you have discovered that your favourite colours do not suit your chosen colour season? In this case, you must try to separate yourself from your 'special' colours. Some women find this difficult because until now they have been quite unconcerned whether their favourite colours suit them or not. Understandably, they will find it difficult to believe these are no longer ideal. Other readers may have problems with identifying their colour type because colours from two quite different season scales appear to suit them well and they cannot decide which suits them best.

The following test will help you to decide finally, and you can also use this to check any decision you may have already made. Please read all the questions relating to the individual colour types and if in doubt look at yourself critically once more in the mirror in daylight.

● If you are making a colour test, go through your wardrobe asking your family to help until you have found items that are in the appropriate colour tone – this could be a towel or something similar. Search around for anything suitable – it is the colour which is important!

● Put a cross in front of every statement with which you agree. Go through all the season types, even if finally you can put a cross against all of the questions.

● In the test, we ask once more about your skin and hair colour, about the way in which you tan in the sun (or not), and about warm or cold colour tones which suit you well or not at all. Please don't be surprised that we have not taken eye colour into account. You probably know yourself how the colour of your eyes subtly changes – depending how the light catches them, the colour of your clothes or even your mood. What is characteristic for the different eye colours is explained on pages 14–21. Otherwise, remember that as far as eye colour is concerned, there are always exceptions to the rule!

● You will probably discover that most of your crosses appear against one particular season type (with only a few against two other types and maybe none against the fourth). The decision is made: your answers indicate your correct season colour type. Despite this, double-check. Make sure you are happy with your answers.

● When you have completed the test think about why you answered as you did. Are you quite certain that you have not made a mistake? Is it possible that one or two single colour nuances on another scale suit you particularly well – but as a cool colour type you can only choose from the cool colour scale and as a warm colour type you can only opt for the second warm scale! In this test, questions are asked about the contrast between warm and cold. You must decide! Do it for yourself – later on, you will be able to instinctively choose the right clothes and the right cosmetics. It will become second nature to you. It will simplify your life.

● The test will help you to decide what suits your natural skin and hair colour as well as your tanned skin. The answers to the questions about colour nuances that particularly suit you – always remembering the colour counselling motto, 'Try it out' – will tell you whether you should stick to just one scale with warm or cold colours.

● Against which colour type have you placed most – ideally all – crosses? Does the result agree with your previous decision?

The Spring type

● Is your skin very delicate, almost transparent?

● Does your complexion have a soft light golden or warm peach-coloured tone? If in doubt compare your skin with other women – do other women have a blue or delicate grey undertone to their skin?

● Do you easily blush? Do you get red blotches quickly if you are excited or under pressure?

● Does your complexion have a natural warm-rose cheek colour (and not a uniform, even ivory tone)?

● Is your hair yellow blonde, flaxen, golden blonde or soft red – yellow-based, not ash-coloured?

● Is your hair a warm light brown or golden brown?

● As a pre-school child did you have really golden blonde hair?

● If you have any red highlights in your hair, is the red shine always there (and not just when the sun shines directly on it)?

● Does your skin tan relatively quickly?

● Does your sun tan have a golden rather than a red tinge (no grey tinge or hazelnut tone)?

● Are your freckles – if you have them – golden brown (not grey-brown)?

Try this out – put a cross beside those statements you agree with:

● Creamy white suits you better than pure white.

● Camel-hair colours and a yellow brown suit you better than grey-brown.

● Salmon colours suit you better than pink.

● Salmon colours suit you better than a strong orange.

● Coral red suits you better than a bluish azalea blue.

● Silver grey suits you better than a metal/anthracite grey.

● Brown tones suit you better than all grey tones.

The Summer type

● Do you sometimes have the feeling that your bare complexion has a cool, almost grey appearance?

● Is your complexion by comparison with others bluish-based rather than golden? (By golden we don't mean yellow.)

● If your skin is darker is it rosy in appearance or a strong, reddish shade?

● Perhaps you feel that none of the previous questions apply to you. If so, is your skin olive?

● Do you tend towards bluish shadows under the eyes?

● Has your hair a clear ash tone (but under no circumstances a yellow tinge)?

● Have you already discovered that silver blonde streaks suit you particularly well?

● Do you often feel your hair colour is mousey and that you should do something about it?

● As a pre-school child were you a light blonde or a true white blonde?

● If you go on holiday to a hot, sunny country do you tan really well?

● When comparing yourself to others, is your suntan grey-brown or hazelnut brown (not golden brown)?

● If you freckle in the sun are your freckles grey-brown or grey-rose (but not golden brown)?

Try this out – put a cross beside those statements you agree with:

● Cool old rose suits you better than all warm salmon tones (they make you look rosier rather than yellow).

● A grey-blue (washed-out, dull blue tone) suits you better than a radiant, clear intensive blue.

● Soft turquoise green suits you better than a yellowish May green.

● Taupe (a subdued grey-brown tone) suits you better than reddish brown and yellow brown colours.

● Grey-brown and very light muddy colours suit you better than camel-hair colours or tile brown.

● Bluish fuchsia red suits you much better than orange red.

● Pink suits you better than apricot.

The Autumn type

● If you have a light complexion is your skin even throughout and ivory-coloured, or is it freckled?

● Have you 'colourless' eye lashes and eye brows?

● When wearing certain types of eye make-up, do your eyes suddenly look enflamed?

● If you have a darker complexion does your skin appear an intensive red gold, like a dark peach or apricot?

● Is your hair red or, more precisely, is it a copper red, rusty red or warm chestnut red (but in no way bluish)?

● If you have brown hair – either light or fairly dark – is it honeyish with always a warm and golden colour?

● Is there absolutely no ash tone in your hair?

● As a child did you have a similar hair colour as today – though now it may be a little darker?

● If you are light-skinned, is it difficult for you to tan? And do you easily burn?

● If you have a dark complexion does your skin tan a Red Indian red without burning badly?

● If freckles develop easily are they an intensive red (red-gold or red-brown)?

Try this out – put a cross beside those statements you agree with:

● Mustard yellow suits you better than buttercup yellow.

● Olive green suits you better than peppermint green.

● Orange suits you better than pink.

● Blackberry suits you better than lilac.

● Anthracite suits you better than chocolate brown.

● Tomato red suits you better than the bluish red of azaleas.

● Petrol (dull blue-green) suits you better than gentian blue.

The Winter type

● If you have a light skin does a bluish tinge show through (similar to porcelain)?

● If you have a darker complexion does your skin have a golden brown tone, or a cool undertone going into olive?

● Do you tend towards strong bluish coloured shadows under your eyes?

● Is there a clear, strong contrast between your hair, skin and eye colour?

● Is your hair dark or even blue-black?

● Is your hair dark brown, middle brown, but always ashy (bluish, with a silver tinge; never golden)?

● If you are blonde, does the typical Winter skin suit you exactly, particularly regarding the strong colour contrasts?

● Have you discovered a few early snow-white hairs?

● If you have a very light complexion how do you tan? Not at all or only a small amount?

● However, if you have a dark complexion do you tan well – a deep much-envied brown?

● Perhaps you belong to the Winter type that freckles: if so, are your freckles grey-brown (never golden brown)?

Try this out – put a cross beside those statements you agree with:

● When wearing black you look radiant (brown clothes make you look sad).

● A clear pink suits you better than old rose.

● Pine green suits you better than olive green, camouflage green or khaki.

● Clear red suits you better than rust or copper.

● Gentian blue suits you better than muddy dove blue.

● Pure snow white suits you better than creamy white.

● Hard marine blue suits you better than soft smoke blue.

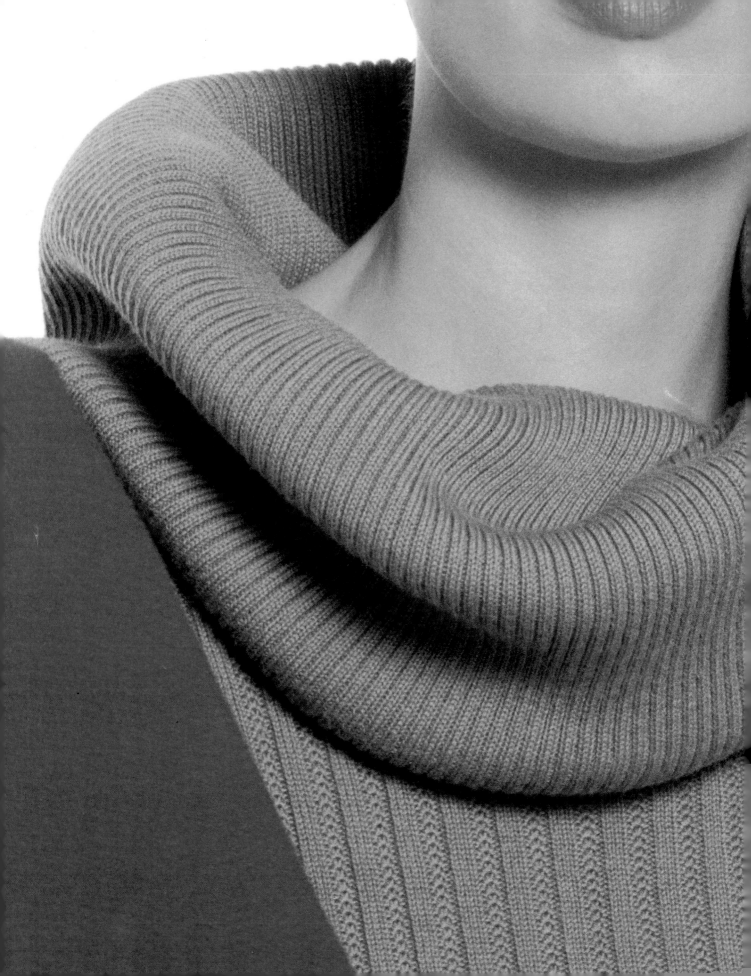

THE COLOURS OF CLOTHES

As you progress you will soon discover something quite remarkable – you do not feel right in colours other than those of your chosen 'season'. Soon you will gladly part with items which at one time you refused to give away and suddenly you find you are immune to the arguments of sales assistants who are selling the fashionable colours of the day. So, given your chosen colour type, how do you look fashionable without looking like everyone else?

Depending on the correct colour tones

Now you know your colour season, you should now know which colours suit you best as well as those you should steer clear of. But continue to take your time and take another look at your colour chart: it is now fairly certain that you will find the colours attractive and harmonious, and that they will suit your personality.

But don't be surprised if you feel there are some colour shades – perhaps a little too powerful or insipid – that you would never wish to wear. If so, you don't have to! But it is always well worth experimenting with colours that up to now you may have rejected. Don't ignore the fact that a particular colour may actually suit you very well, even though you may never have realised it before! Colour counselling is about opening up your ideas; it's about freedom.

If you now rummage through your wardrobe you will almost certainly discover that you have already instinctively bought some of your clothes in the right colours. It is well worth taking the time to sort through your clothes and take out those items which you now know are really the wrong colours for you. You may never enjoy wearing them now so why not take them to a charity shop, swop them with a friend or maybe alter them in some way?

Take care when sorting through your clothes in the 'wrong' colours – some things can be saved.

Perhaps some of the clothes to which you are so attached can be dyed? Of course, they may not match exactly the colour on your chart but an approximation will do just as well. It is sometimes enough if, say, Summer and Winter types dye their yellow and salmon coloured blouses a cool blue; Spring and Autumn women could dye their cool, light clothes with a warm yellowish tone. If you are dyeing one or two pieces together in the washing machine remember you may get different results depending on the material dyed – but all the colours should harmonise.

You do not need to be quite so merciless when sorting out skirts and trousers (and other items which are not worn next to the face). These items can be combined in different ways. You must not be too rigid and dogmatic – no one expects you to throw out all your favourite things in one fell swoop! Keep on wearing them for as long as you feel 'right' in them. But soon you will begin to notice you are taking an increased interest in 'your' colours and that clothes in other colours are no longer so attractive to you. Your imagination is stimulated – which blouse, which scarf and which accessories bring a new touch and identity to your favourite sweater?

Knowing your colour type makes buying clothes that much easier.

You will soon find that shopping has become much easier. After a while you will automatically reject those clothes in colours which do not suit you, concentrating on those which do. Of course, you know what suits you best – even when the sales person argues that another colour is particularly fashionable and, of course, you can wear it! Under no circumstances forget the following tips when you are spending your hard earned money on new clothes.

● Always keep your colour chart in your handbag and use it to make comparisons in daylight with the item you are considering buying. In most shops the lighting is purposely flattering and diffuse and colours are rarely true, while in some changing cubicles harsh neon lighting distorts colour in a similar way.

● Do not be too disappointed if you cannot find the exact colour shades that you have on your charts. It is impossible, as textile colours will always have a different appearance when compared with colours printed on paper – the texture is different and therefore reflects light differently. Imagine the colour blue in silk, linen, leather, satin and tweed: sometimes the blue will appear radiant and intense, at other times dull and more subdued ...

The important thing is that the colour tone you have chosen harmonises with your colour chart. For example, check that the blue of a dress falls within the blue tones on your chart, that it is a cool or a clearly warm colour, and that it does not differ too greatly in intensity from those on the chart.

● Sometimes it is not easy to determine whether a colour is really cold or warm. A blouse in subdued red, for example, appears to be a typically cool Summer colour: then you wonder – is it a softer, warmer Spring red?

In such a situation you can do only one thing. Compare the blouse in daylight with other red items in the shop as only a direct comparison will help you to decide.

● You also now know it is possible that colours, other than those on your own chart, may suit you well. For example, as a Summer type you can wear the dark blue of Winter or as Spring you may be able to wear Autumn's salmon tones. Lucky you! If you are a 'mixed type' and like these colours then wear them. However, there is one thing you should never do; as a cool Summer and Winter woman, never wear a colour from the warm ranges. Or as a Spring or Autumn woman who finds warm colours suit her, never choose the cooler colours.

After the initial enthusiasm wears off, such choices will become automatic and you will instinctively accept that it is a question of looking as good as you possibly can. You have arrived!

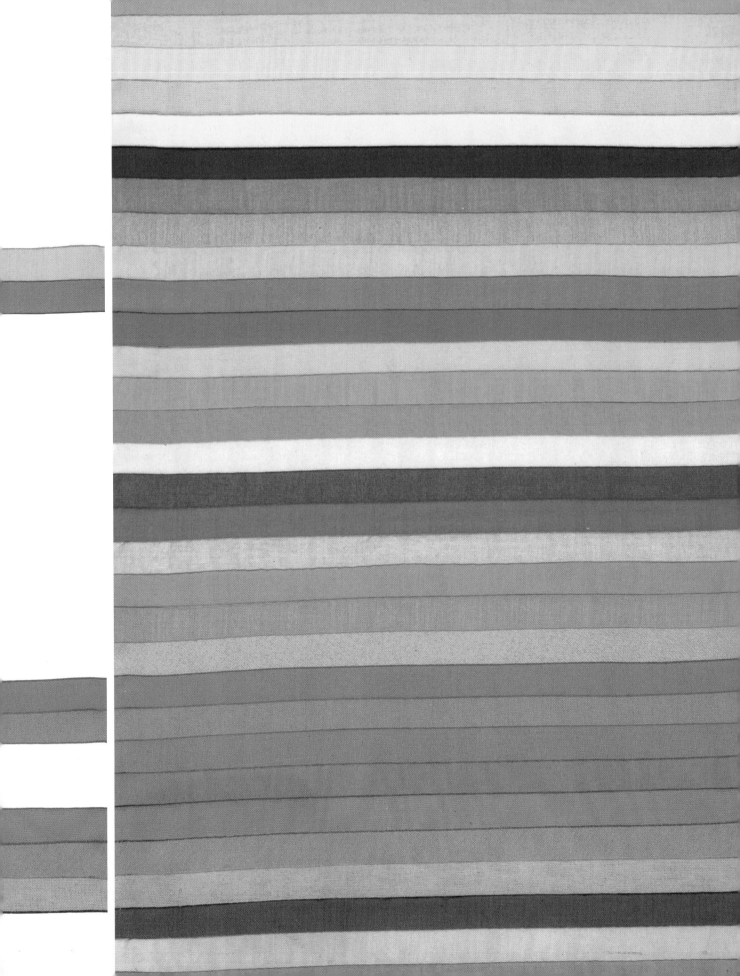

The prettiest colours for the Spring type

Light and clear are the ideal colours for the Spring woman – some colours are delicate, others radiate intensely. Mousey tones make the Spring type look uninteresting. This is also true of colours that are too strong or with nuances that are too dark – they overwhelm Spring's fine complexion. Despite this, Spring women can wear the whole range of colours on their palette. For example, May green, apple green, lime green ... indeed every green that looks as though it is flooded with sunshine. And, of course, warm, full yellows. All delicate rose and red tones tinged with yellow suit the Spring type well – peach, apricot, salmon and warm coral red. Pink on the other hand, leaves women of this type looking insipid, and the bluish red of Summer makes them look pale and boring. Spring types with a creamy soft or lightly tanned complexion look serene in woollen white, golden camel-hair tones and the soft brown of milk chocolate – blouse and blazer look excellent when matched tone by tone with each other and suit both hair and skin. As the skin of the Spring type usually tans a light golden brown, many Spring women make the fatal mistake of accentuating their tan with pure white clothes. But this does not leave them looking crisp and brown; it has a parchment effect, giving a much older look. For a more flattering effect, Spring types should choose a warm brown and gold-beige or, for contrast, a clear aquamarine blue or soft light turquoise which accentuates the tan and is much more harmonious. Creamy eggshell whites suit the complexion of the Spring type much better than a hard, bright white. Black is taboo (except of course, for small accessories which bring out the radiance of other colours); the darkest colours which suit Spring are a relatively light marine blue, soft violet and warm chocolate brown. And should a Spring woman particularly wish to wear grey – normally a colour they should leave well alone! – a gentle silver grey is the best choice.

Photo left: a range of radiant and clear tones is available to the Spring type - mousey tones should be avoided. If you are beginning to build a basic wardrobe we would recommend three colours – the extended coloured strips – light grey-blue tones, apricot in all colour options and soft camel-hair colours.

Basic colour: grey-blue

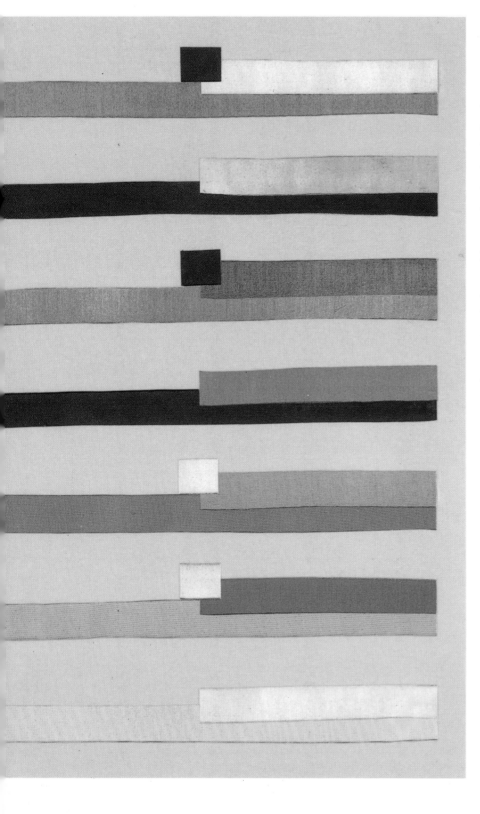

Light blue with a hint of grey is a relatively neutral colour and an excellent choice for the Spring type. For this reason we would advise making this soft blue the base for your wardrobe: it is an easy colour to mix 'n' match. The colour chart on the left illustrates this well – ochre, white and brown; brown and beige; three types of violet nuances; violet and rose-wood; lobster red; turquoise and white; silver grey, royal blue and a dab of yellow, and May green and white all co-ordinate perfectly. All other colours in the Spring range of course suit just as well!

Photo right: Spring's ideal combination of two basic wardrobe colours – the suit in light blue, the coat in camel–hair colour. Pretty with it: a shiny white blouse

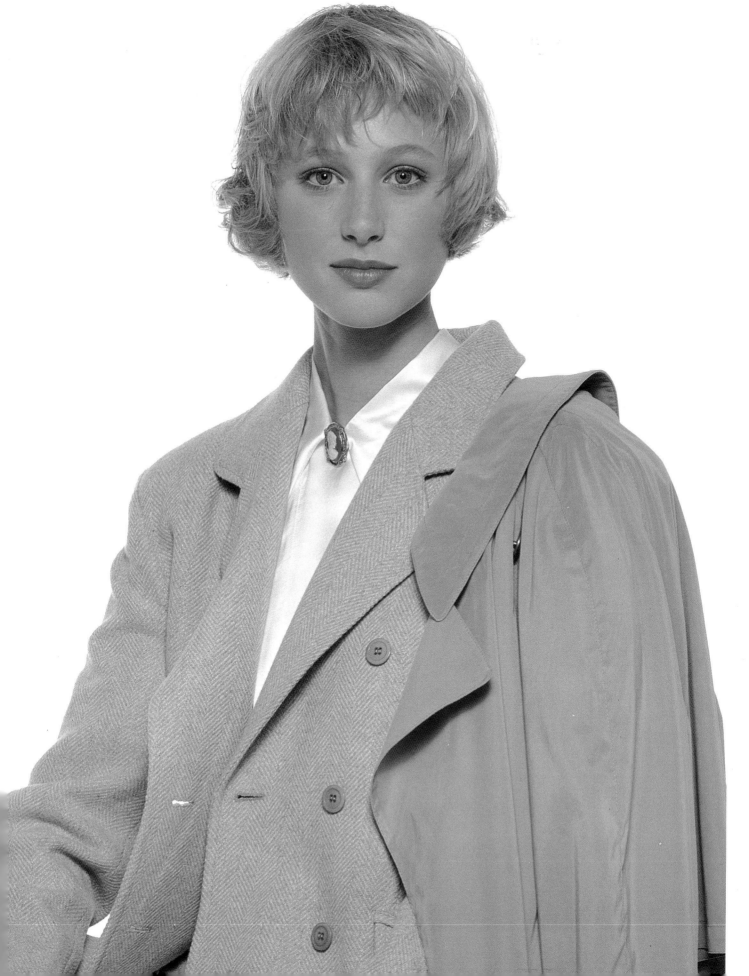

Basic colour: apricot

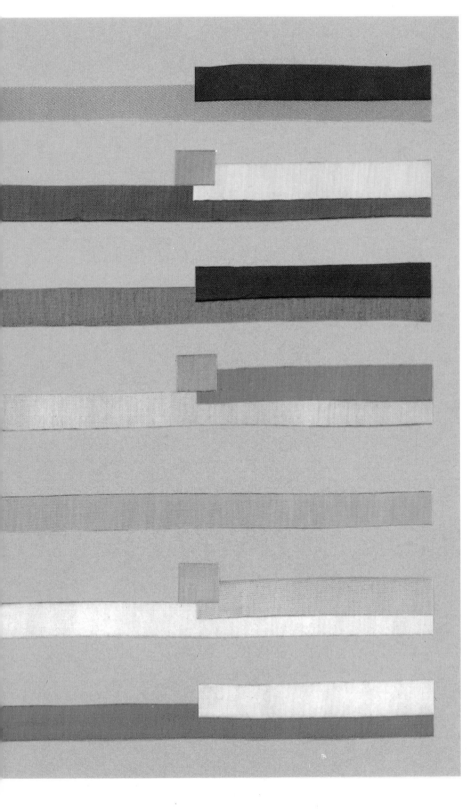

Apricot as the basic colour – now this is unusual. Only Spring types can afford this extravagance and, as such, they should consider it from time to time! Anyone not wishing to make apricot her basic colour, can choose it as the dominant second colour (see photo right). Again, on the left we illustrate a series of colour combinations which highlight apricot to a most brilliant effect: camel-hair colours and brown; light brown, beige and a dab of rosewood; light and dark violet; grey-blue, royal blue and ochre; pure sky blue; white, silver-grey and green, and red and white.

Photo right: apricot as the dominant combination colour. Its freshness is subdued by the camel-hair colour and looks good when worn with a normally unsuitable black skirt.

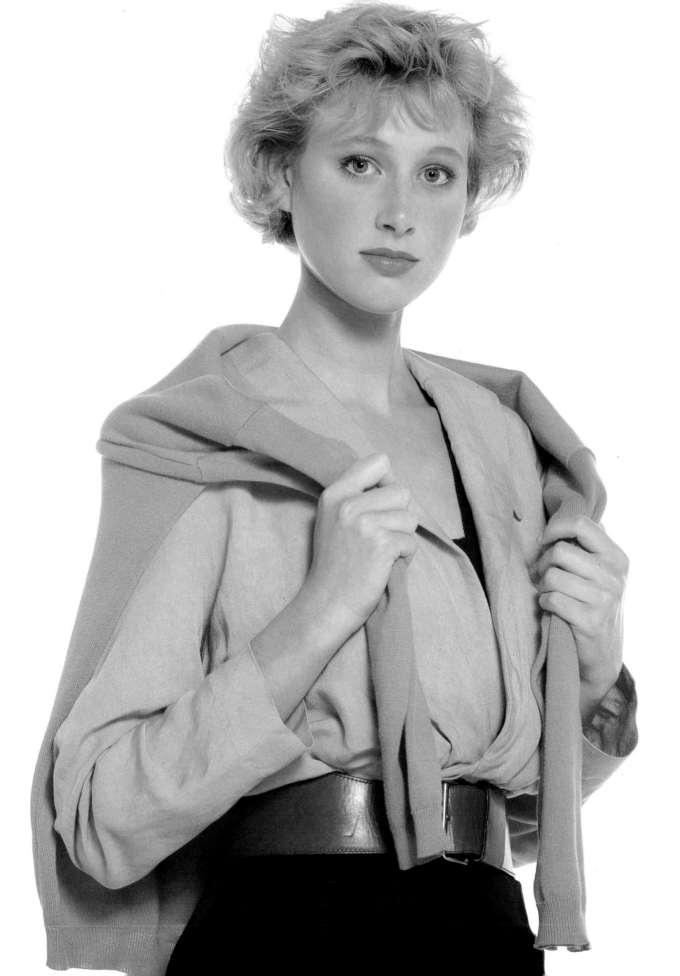

Basic colour: camel-hair

L ight, soft camel-hair colours flatter Spring types but make other women look boring. Camel-hair colours in almost all shades, in light green nuances, in golden and light browns, are ideal as a basic wardrobe colour. As a combination colour, all colours in the Spring range are suitable for co-ordinating with camel-hair shades; particularly good are those printed on the left – grey-blue and violet; royal blue, beige brown and violet; brown and ochre; yellow, red and white; white and green; May green and lobster red, lobster red, sky blue and red.

Photo right: the cape coat in Spring's basic camel-hair colour has a green hint and co-ordinates well with the other Spring colours worn, sky blue and violet (in skirt).

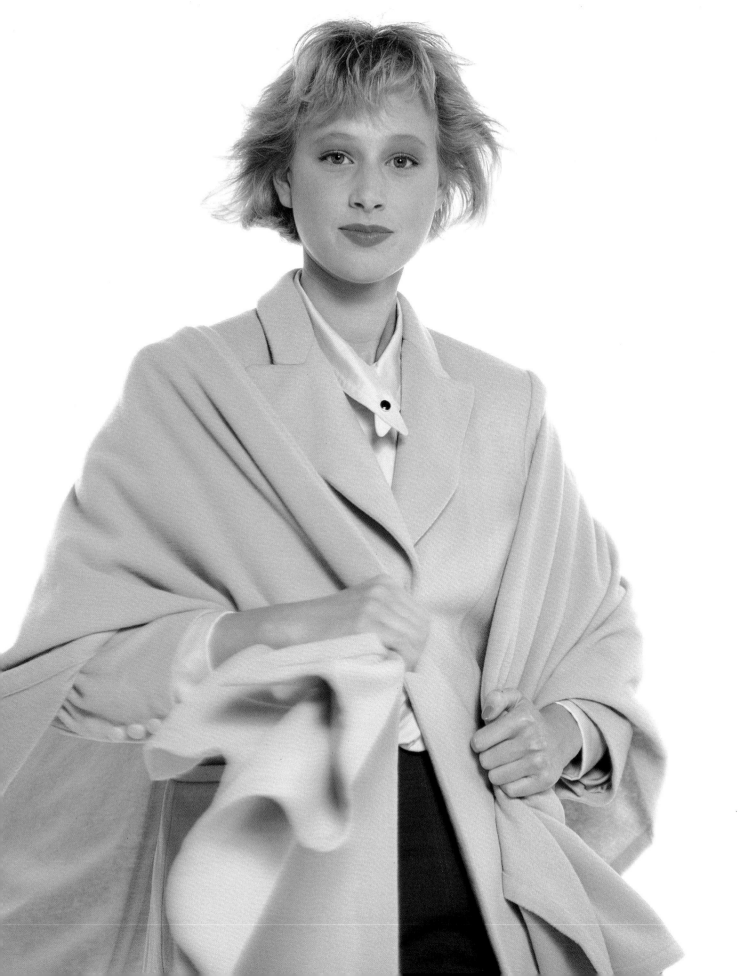

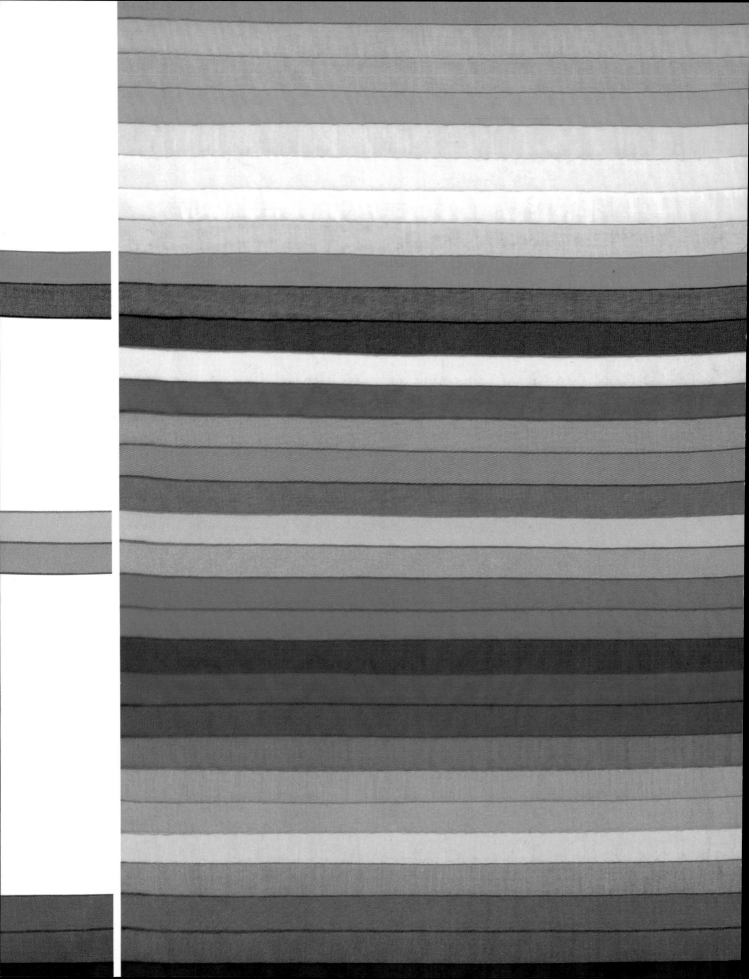

The best colours for the Summer type

Say goodbye to all those dazzling colours! Perhaps you already instinctively know that a bikini in neon green, bright blue or tomato red does not suit you – although it may be the height of fashion – and, if worn with a tan, give you a positively ageing lilac tinge! Summer types look terrific in soft, aristocratic-looking colour tones. Have a look at your colour chart – almost all of the colour tones look as if they have been mixed with grey, powdery rose or washed-out blue. This is because all these subtle colours harmonise perfectly with the blue undertone of the skin and the silver ashy hair of Summer types. Colours which leave other types looking weak, liven up Summer women; nearly all pastel tones suit you just as long as they have the soft blue or grey undertone. No yellow, salmon pink, apricot or peach please!

Pink, however, flatters the Summer type lending a lighter or fresher appeal, depending whether you are pale-skinned or have a more intensive skin colour. And do you think red doesn't suit you? Imagine a fruit stall: the red of the tomato is too yellow; raspberry red on the other hand (a light bluish red) is exactly right for you, as is the red seen inside a cut water melon! Carrot red should be avoided at all costs, but in its place you can choose the full (bluish) red of ripe cherries and, if you like a dark red, wine red is perfect. Every smokey blue suits you well (you are just the right type for stone-washed jeans!) as well as all bluish greens from turquoise to fairly dark tones. But be careful with yellow! The best shade for you is a single, quite delicate, cool lemon yellow. Plain, unpatterned white and black can only rarely be worn by Summer types – a more harmonious effect is achieved by opting for a rosy, cool or soft grey toned white; as for dark colours, Summer types look best in a smokey navy-blue or a brown with a rose or grey tinge.

Photo left: wonderfully cool and subdued is the effect of the colour chart for Summer types. No glaring colours can be seen; instead, smokey pastel nuances are preferred. Highlighted are three colour suggestions for Summer's basic wardrobe (the colours of the extended strips) – subdued blue tones; cool, rather grey-based brown tones, and old to lilac rose.

Basic colour: dark blue

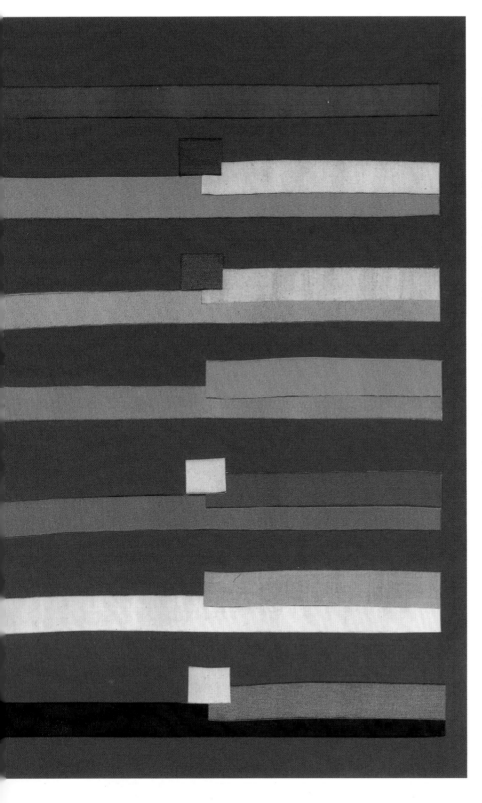

Subdued blue – never brilliant or shrill! – is always right for the Summer type and an ideal colour for a basic wardrobe. According to personal taste, it can be a dull denim blue, smokey navy-blue or a red-tinged plum blue. Every one of these blues harmonises with the combinations printed left: a pure bluish summer red; green, white and a spot of red; grey, light rose and brown; pink and blue-green; denim blue, red and white; vanilla yellow and light blue, and dark brown, lilac and vanilla yellow.

Photo right: Dark blue, perhaps with a light red tinge, as a basic colour for the Summer type's wardrobe. Perfectly co-ordinated are blue-tinged summer reds.

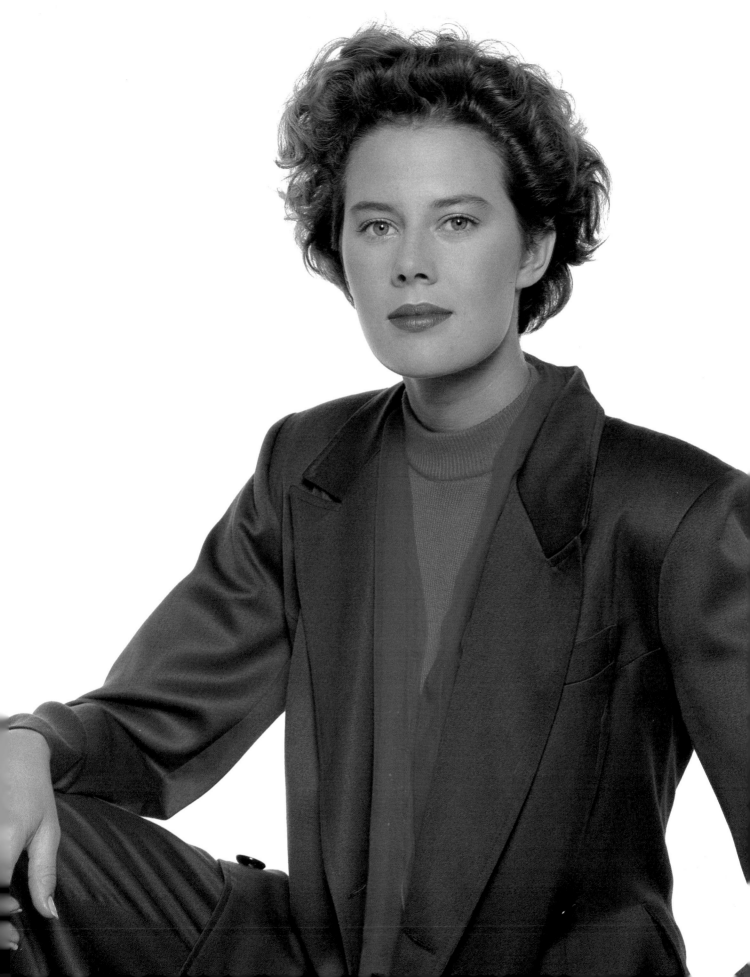

Basic colour: brown

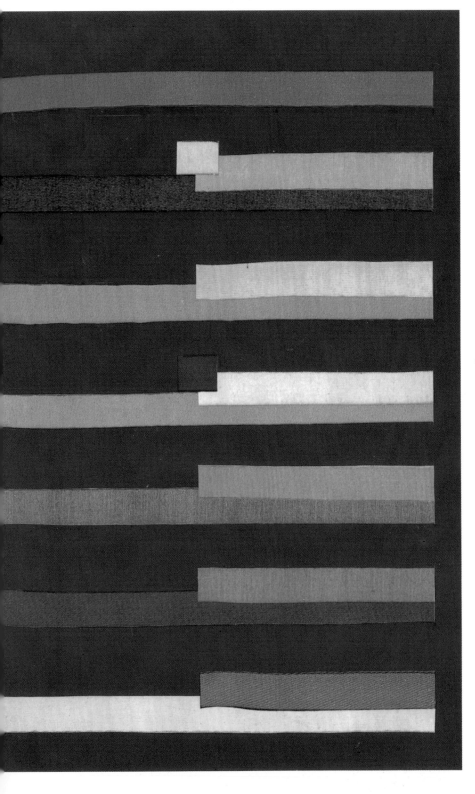

Summer types can wear brown very well. But be careful: a 'warm' brown has a deadening effect – choose one which is shot through with a touch of grey or tinged a reddish blue. Think of plain chocolate which harmonises with all Summer's colours. Illustrated left, are the best colours for Summer's basic brown: jeans-blue; smokey blue with light green and white; dark with light emerald; grey with white and red; taupe with rose; lilac with old rose, and yellow with violet.

Photo right: brown as a basic colour for the Summer type can look very elegant, but needs at least one other powerful colour. Here, denim blue shirt and jeans balance the strong brown.

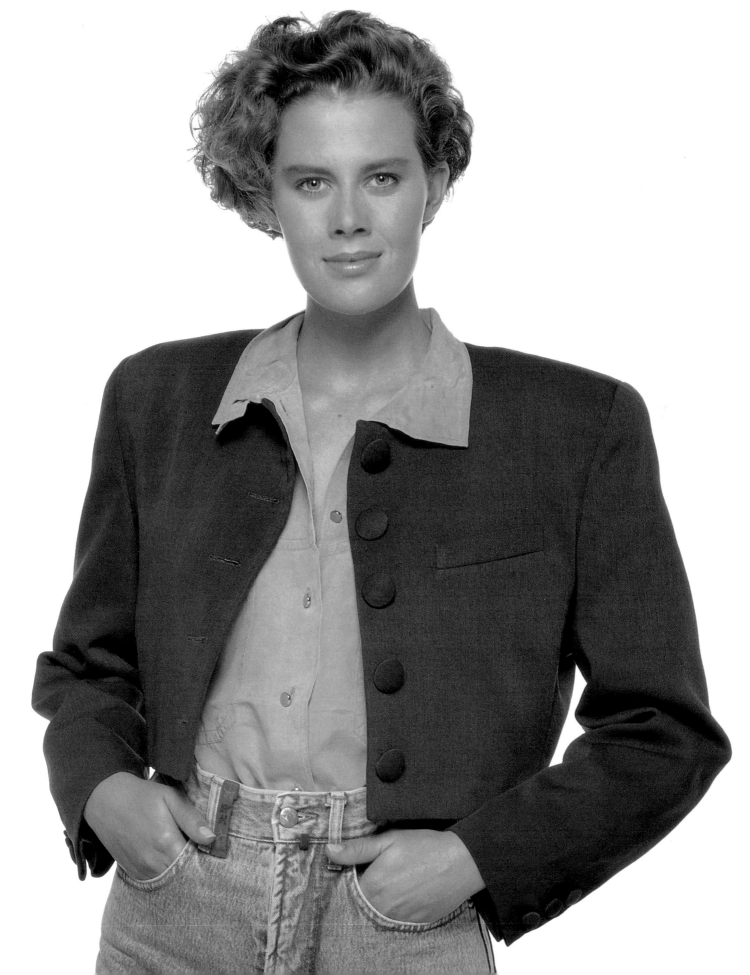

Basic colour: lilac rose

A flattering, soft grey, lilac rose can certainly be considered as a basic colour for the Summer type, but those who find the colour too 'sickly' for major wardrobe items might prefer to use it more sparingly. But remember – lilac rose needs one or more combination colours.

A few suggestions are shown, left: pure lavender; dark blue with pink; summer red with dark brown; brown with light brown and a touch of dark blue; mid-brown with ivory white; silver grey with yellow and denim blue, and dark and light emerald with smokey blue.

Photo right: parka-style jacket in lilac rose as a base for a Summer wardrobe, harmonizing with and 'lifted' by the dark lavender trousers.

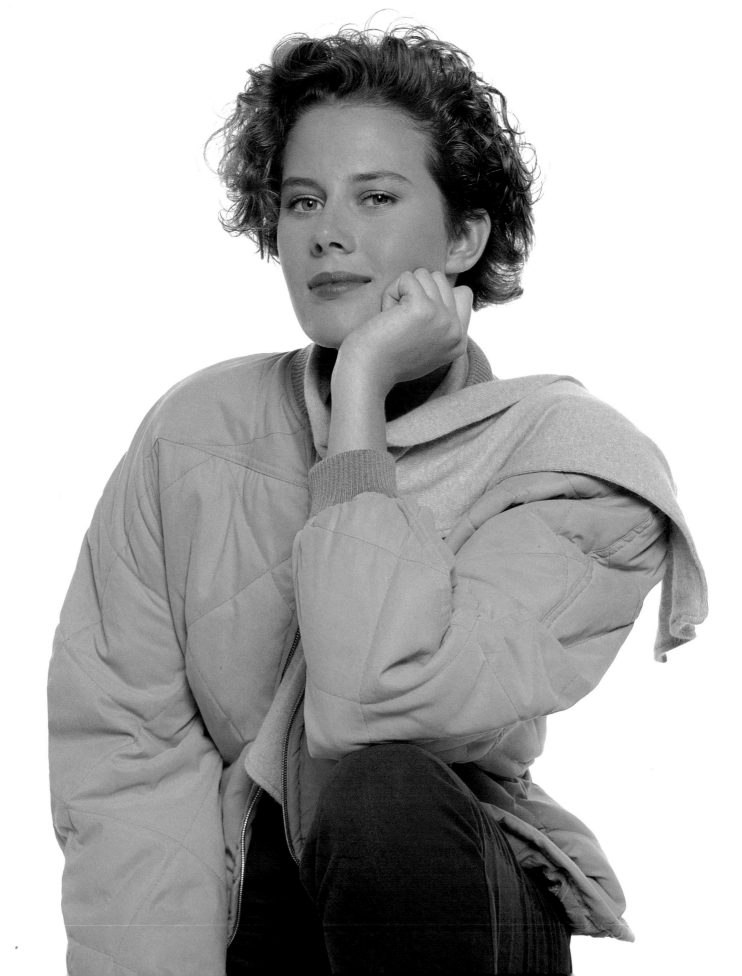

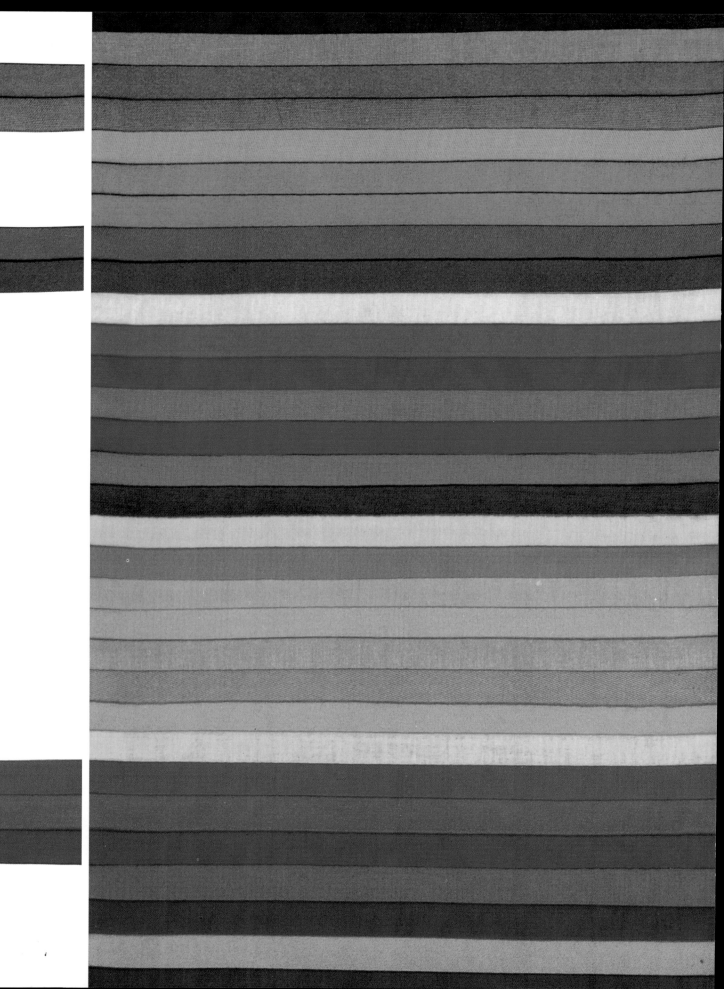

Warm colours for the Autumn type

Autumn colours are wonderfully indulgent – warm, earthy, with a wisp of gold, or clear, full and rich – and the choice depends on whether the Autumn woman has a light, ivory skin or a more lively, peach-coloured complexion. Ideal for all Autumn types are warm brown tones from light champagne and gold beige through warm, full rust to the darkest chocolate brown. All golden or warm red-brown shades complement the Autumn type very well, bringing a healthy radiance to her skin. She must be more careful with cool grey-browns which tend to make her look anaemic and pale. Even the lively blue-green of Summer (to which unfortunately many Autumn types feel attracted) should be carefully considered as it could make her look gaudy. However, the Autumn woman looks particularly attractive in green tones which harmonise perfectly with her colouring; these include a sunny pea-green through to olive; light and powerful khaki through to petrol; Russian green, and dark pine green. Although slightly blue, a graceful, milky jade green, full, dark turquoise and all red-blue tones (plum blue to bluish violet) also suit the Autumn type. On a surprising note – Autumn women are the only ones who look good wearing a full, brilliant orange, but at all costs they should avoid all pink tones!

The rose and red shades which suit the Autumn woman are always the warmer tones – salmon and apricot rose, poppy red, tomato red and copper red. 'Difficult' colours like mustard yellow and a reddish maize yellow seem to have been made exclusively for Autumn women, allowing them to blossom while lending a sickly air to other types! Should you be an Autumn type try to steer clear of black and pure white – dark chocolate brown and a creamy, ivory white suit you much better.

Photo left: khaki tones, bluish green and a still, warm petrol, as well as red-brown and gold rust are ideal colours for the basic wardrobe of Autumn types (see the extended colour strips far left in the illustration). These groups harmonise with all the warm, Autumn colours on the chart.

Basic colour: petrol

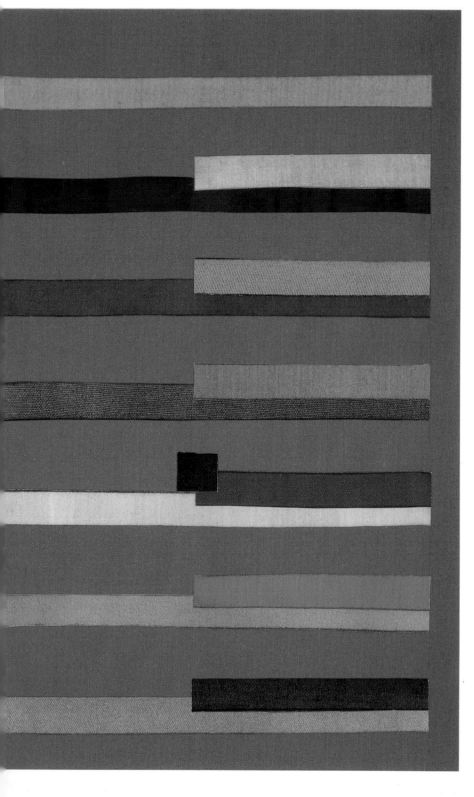

Autumn types whose favourite colour is blue will find blue-green petrol a distinctive and extremely attractive colour for their basic wardrobe. Petrol is a bold colour and should be combined with similarly strong and lively colours. On the chart on the left for example it co-ordinates well with a cheeky orange; brown and peach; rust red and slate green; khaki and brass; creamy white, blackberry red and a touch of brown; light brown and tomato red, and with brass and plum blue.

Photo right: illustrating how petrol is a much more attractive basic wardrobe colour for the Autumn woman (instead of the usual navy-blue), but one which demands strong combination colours, such as this orange wrap-over blouse.

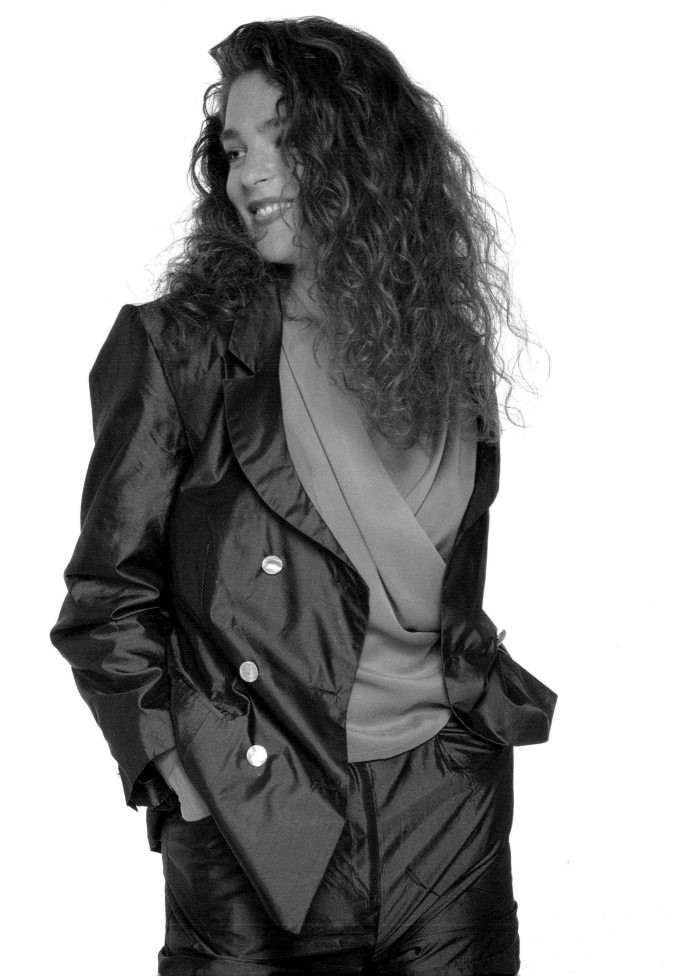

Basic colour: khaki

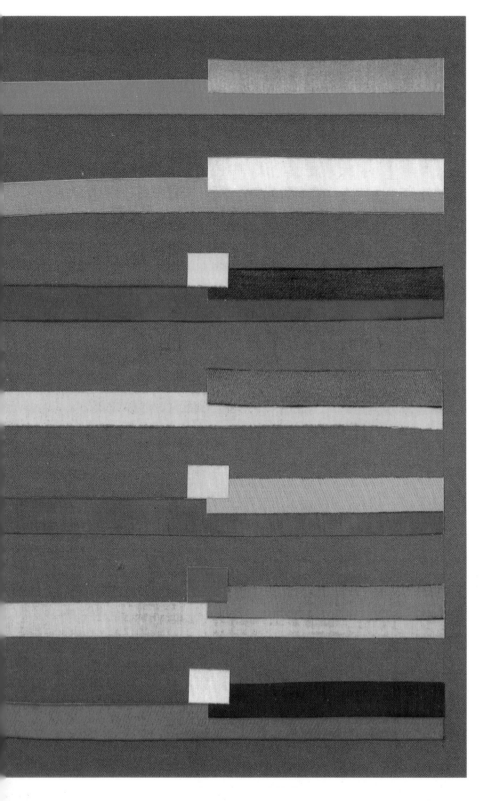

The many subdued shades between green and brown – all described as khaki – suit the Autumn woman well and are excellent as her basic wardrobe colour. Khaki is a classic, reserved colour which brings a brilliance to Autumn's complexion and hair colouring.

Illustrated left is a range of colours from Autumn's colour palette which co-ordinate well with khaki: tomato red and brass; lobster red and creamy white; blackberry red, plum blue and a spot of golden yellow; golden yellow and petrol; rust, slate green and peach colours; peach colours, bluish violet and red, and red brown and a little creamy white.

Photo right: Khaki, whether dark as the spotted sweater or quite light as the trousers, is a good basic colour for Autumn's wardrobe. It co-ordinates with – and demands – strong combination colours such as orange, golden yellow and red.

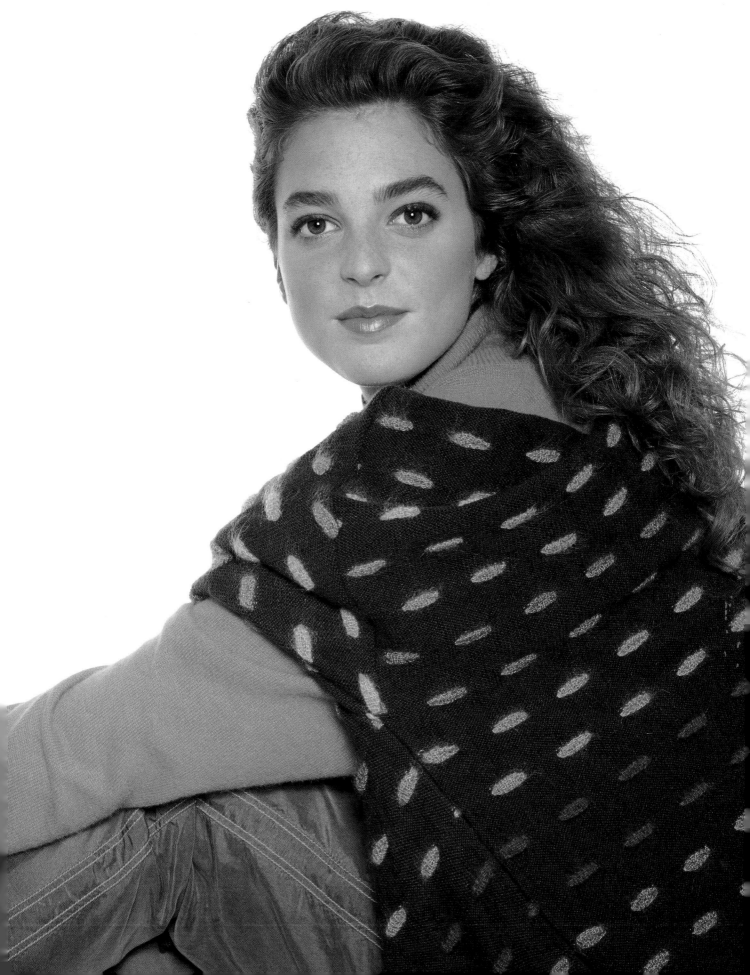

Basic colour: rust brown

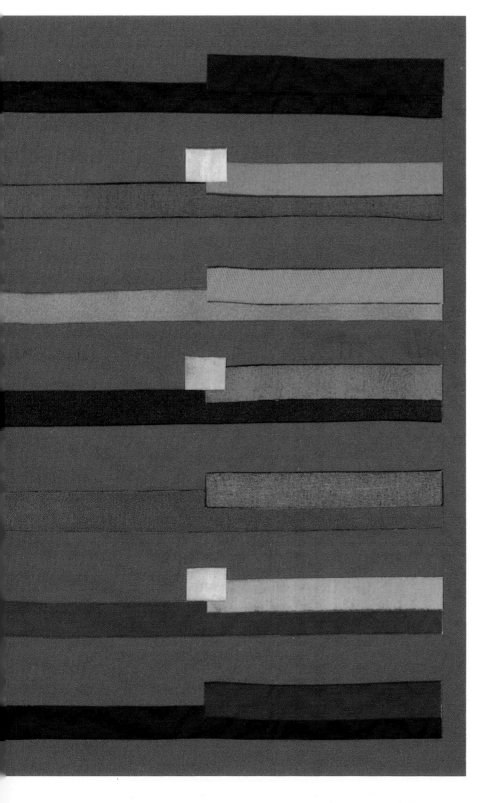

Rust brown is a colour which suits most Autumn types best of all. It harmonises with their honey-coloured hair; it complements a light ivory complexion as well as peach-coloured skins, and it combines wonderfully well with many other Autumn colours. Shown left a few examples: plum blue with brown; bluish violet with a lot of orange and a little creamy white; camel-hair with slate green; dark and light petrol with peach; pine green with moss green; red with yellow and a little creamy white, and brown with blackberry red.

Photo right: rust brown is Autumn's best basic wardrobe colour and one which many women will instinctively choose. The rich rust red of the jacket is perfectly complemented by the deep red of the trousers and the scarf's violet shade.

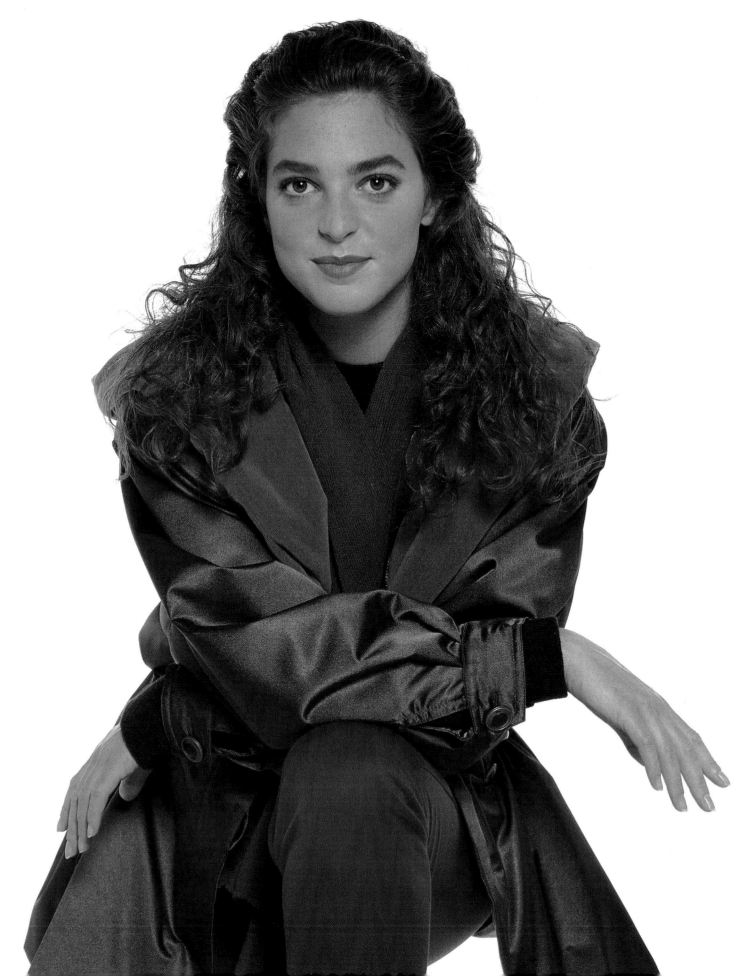

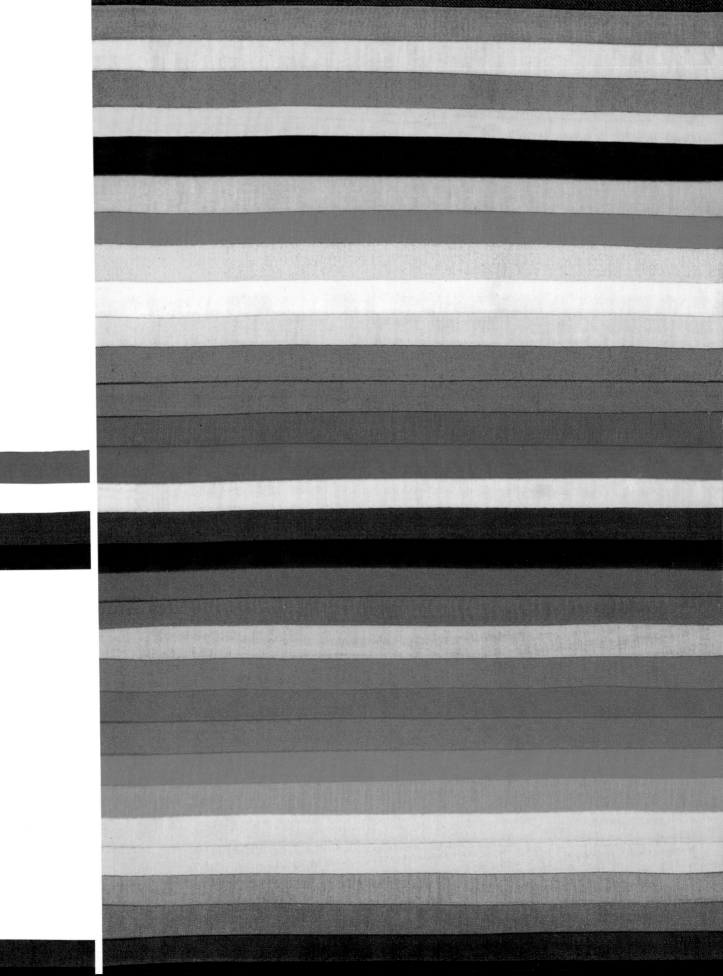

Contrast for the Winter type

Take a minute to look at the colour chart on the left – its colours are the clearest and coolest of all. Cool and clear like the natural colours of the Winter type. These colours, which so far we have been avoiding, are right for Winter women: for example, snow white and a deep black look particularly good.

Winter types thrive on contrasts – between their skin and hair colour as well as between the iris and whites of their eyes. And many Winter types already instinctively know cool colours are right for them. Unfortunately, others seem to have a lifelong fatal preference for warm, earthy autumn colours which, with their black-brown hair and maybe an olive-toned skin, shows how a misdiagnosis is easily made! Warm, earthy colours make Winter women look yellow. Better for them are the intense ruby and scarlet reds – no tomato please – powerful pinks and azaleas as well as a cool lilac and dark violet. If a Winter type likes green it should be a clear, strong green tone not washed-out, milky or yellow greens and if choosing a brown tone then please choose only the darkest and coolest – like a deep, plain chocolate. And the Winter woman is the only type who can wear a deep powerful blue – bright blue, gentian blue, Caribbean blue or similar – it looks terrific and balances Winter's strong contrasts.

An additional word about Winter's light colours: if you are a more delicate Winter type with a passion for pastel colours – try them! On your chart you will find many pastel shades, but each one – from grey through rose to creamy yellow – are all icy clear, very distinct and really quite light.

Photo left: Black suits all Winter types – whether or not it is fashionable – and together with anthracite grey is an ideal basic colour for a Winter's wardrobe. Dramatic cherry red is also a suitable base colour but for those Winter women looking for a more conventional colour around which to base their wardrobes, night blue or navy-blue may be preferred (see also the extended colour strips).

Basic colour: black

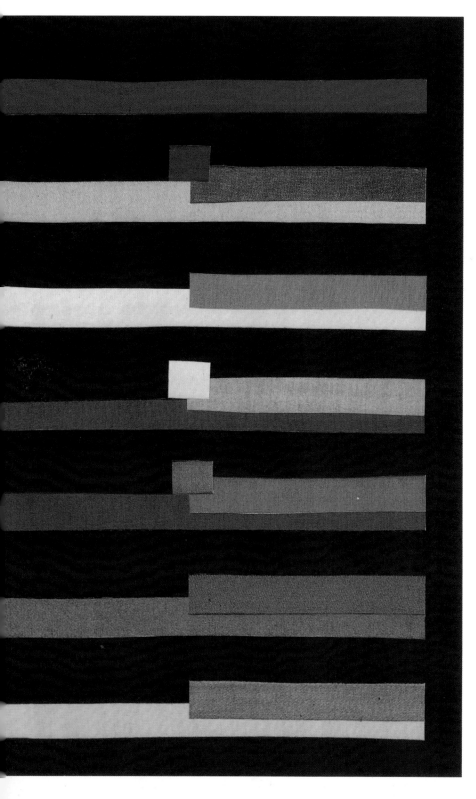

Black is the Winter type's ideal colour for a basic wardrobe: these women are the only ones for which black – whether on its own or combined with other colours – is really suitable. In addition, black strengthens the effect of all the other Winter colours, something else the Winter type carries off spectactularly well. Shown left is the range of Winter colour combinations to be considered with black: pure, strong pink; yellow with grey and red; ice yellow with rose; lilac, pale lilac and ice yellow; indigo with orange and grey; bottle green with azure, and ice green with jade green.

Photo right: black is a terrific basic colour for Winter's wardrobe for both daytime or evening. It is especially effective when worn here with a strong pink.

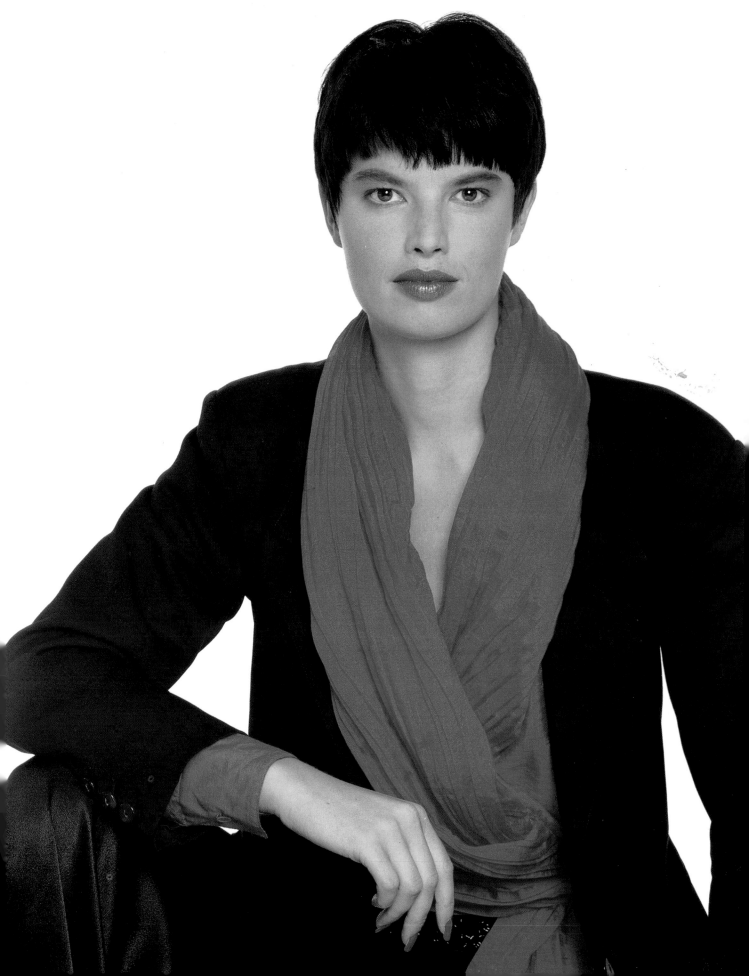

Basic colour: night blue

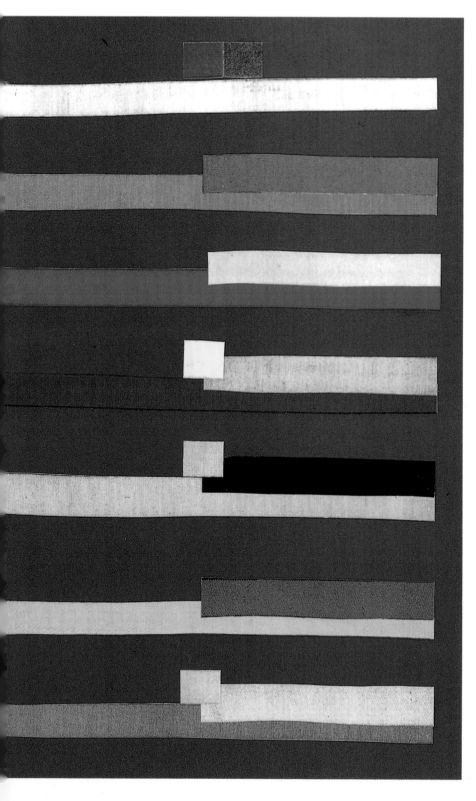

Night blue is an ideal basic colour for the Winter woman's wardrobe; it is easier than black, suits them well and in combination with nearly all of the other Winter colours, is stunningly effective. Shown left are a few suggestions for night blue colour combinations: the red-white-green trio (used effectively in photo opposite); pink with pine green; classical red and white; dark and light lilac with a touch of yellow; icy peach with dark brown and silver grey; fresh May green with emerald, and silver grey with strong yellow and a touch of icy rose.

Photo right: a blazer in a basic night blue colour is timeless when sportily combined with white trousers, navy-blue stripes and an eye-catching belt with red, green and white colour touches.

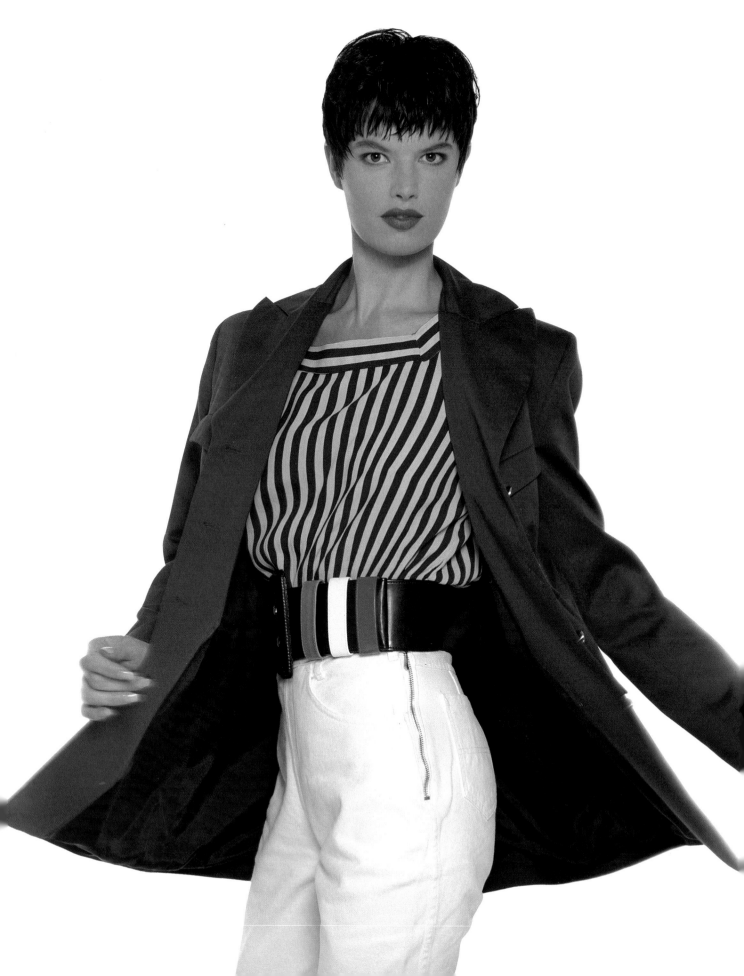

Basic colour: red

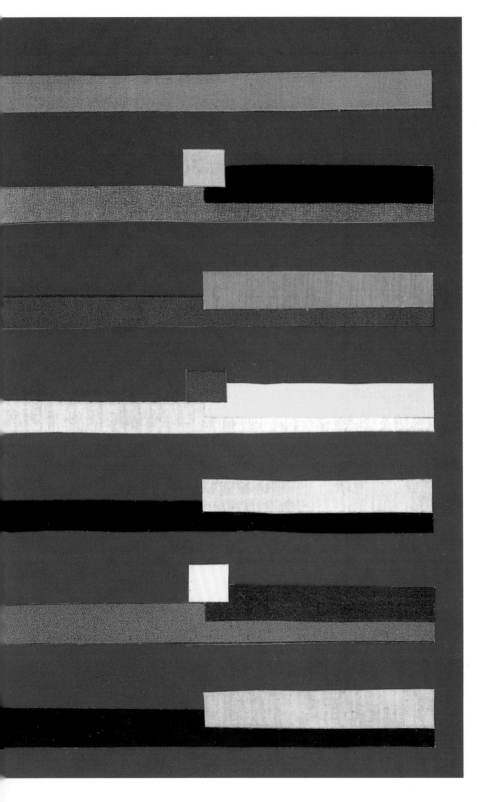

Only Winter types can wear bright red as the basic wardrobe colour because only their colouring has the strength to carry it. The delicate natural colours of the Spring and Summer types can be easily overwhelmed by large areas of red and Autumn women run the danger of looking cheap in red. Only the Winter woman looks good in red as a basic colour and even then she can wear it with equally strong colours (see left). For example with green; grey, black and ice blue; lilac and rose; white, yellow and lilac; black and silver grey; azure, dark blue and ice yellow, and with black-brown and sand colours.

Photo right: brilliant red as a basic colour is very striking and suitable only for the Winter woman. Red should always be balanced with another strong colour, in this case, green.

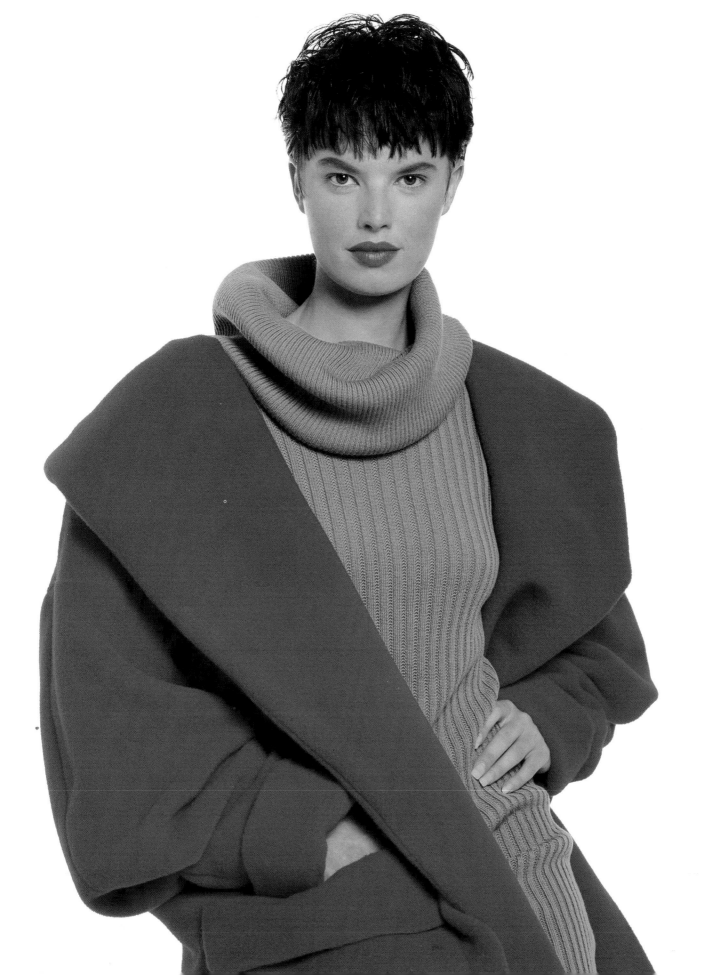

Just a word about white

White is special. You may be convinced that it suits you or perhaps you feel it is not right for you? Don't worry: white is a 'difficult' colour and choosing the right one is tricky.

There are lots of white shades – the white of porcelain is different to that of enamel and the white of a lily is different to that of a rose. Even such a common description as 'blossom white' is unclear – which blossom is meant? Are salt, bleached flour and polished rice all the same white? Even when we say 'white as snow', the meaning is not always clear; the snow after a frosty night is a different colour to that of freshly fallen snow; impacted snow looks quite different to snow which is just about to melt. And is a white sandy beach really white?

White is full of symbolism. It stands for innocence and purity as well as for perfection and brightness. The Pope's robe is white, as is a sterile hospital room; a bride's dress is white; doctors and laboratory assistants wear white. It is thought to be a 'clean' colour. No wonder that some women like wearing white blouses – after all, white symbolises what the advertising slogans call 'appetisingly fresh' and 'clean and pure'. According to common belief, white makes everything look friendlier, lighter and appetising.

In contrast however, white clothes can look harder, more boring or even grubby. It all depends on which tone of white is worn.

There are countless nuances of white – it is important to distinguish between cold or warm tones.

Among the countless white variations we can make a distinction between two large groups – the 'cold' and the 'warm' white tones.

For example, pure white has a cold effect. Think of some types of paper or whitewash, also milky white, putty white and the clean white of freshly fallen snow. A cold effect is also produced by white with a tinge of grey as well as the bluish shimmering white of porcelain.

The warm whites include the whiteness of wool, the pale yellow white of cream, and the soft shades of eggshell and ivory white.

If you cannot immediately decide which white is right for you – whether it is 'cool' or 'warm' – place a piece of typing paper next to it – does the fabric look warmer and yellower? Or is it a little greyer and cooler?

By now you should be fully developing your eye for colour and you should find it becoming easier to make your choices. But when considering white, there are still some important rules:

● Generally speaking, those women who look best in cooler colours – Summer and Winter – can only wear a cool white; those women who look best in warmer colours – Spring and Autumn – should only wear warm whites.

● But remember your individuality: anyone with a very light complexion with light eyes and light hair, can appear boring and even paler in white – whether cool or warm. In this case, pastel colours are better.

● Anyone who tans quickly and deeply (Spring, for example) or who has a natural, brownish complexion (Autumn) tends to over-emphasise a tan when wearing a brilliant, cool white. This produces a strong contrast: the skin looks leathery and burned, and loses its golden brown shimmer. The white is too harsh.

● For anyone who is uncertain about which white really suits them, a wool white can be worn well by every woman. Wool white is a warm white – a soft, light, creamy white colour. It is not a yellow white. Designers are fond of this soft neutral and in the fashion world it is sometimes called 'winter white'. This has nothing to do with our Winter colour type.

● Continue to experiment with your whites. And remember – it is generally true that only the Winter woman can wear a pure, cool white; Spring types look best in a soft wool white; Summer women suit a blue milk white, and Autumn looks best in a light yellow, creamy white.

... and about patterns

Whether a sweater, dress or trousers, almost every woman has a few patterned items in her wardrobe. Or she has seen something in a pattern which she is very keen to buy. But as far as colour is concerned patterns are not easy to assess: maybe a small check has just two colours; or maybe ten or more different colours? A paisley pattern has a green-blue effect, but when you look more closely you will see also violet, brown and even some gold. So which charts should you use as a reference?

If you choose a patterned item - whether a large sweater design or smaller flowers on a summer skirt - you should consider the following:

● What is the basic colour in the pattern?

● Does the character of the pattern suit your colour type and your body proportions?

Look at the item from a distance. What is the general impression? Which colour tone dominates? Does this harmonise with your colour chart?

If you see one or two subsidiary patterns, don't worry. As long as they are subtle and are not prominent they shouldn't be a problem. But be very careful with a conspicuous, evenly coloured pattern. For example, a sweater with a large knitted picture on the front may be the right background colour for you - but what about the coloured picture? Does the whole effect swamp you?

Your colour chart should give you some help with the type of pattern which suits you. Contrasting strong, even colours suit the Winter type (but would overwhelm Spring women). Spring types suit clear and delicate patterns while blurred and powdery patterns are best for Summer types. Finally, for Autumn women soft, non-contrasting patterns are the preferred choices.

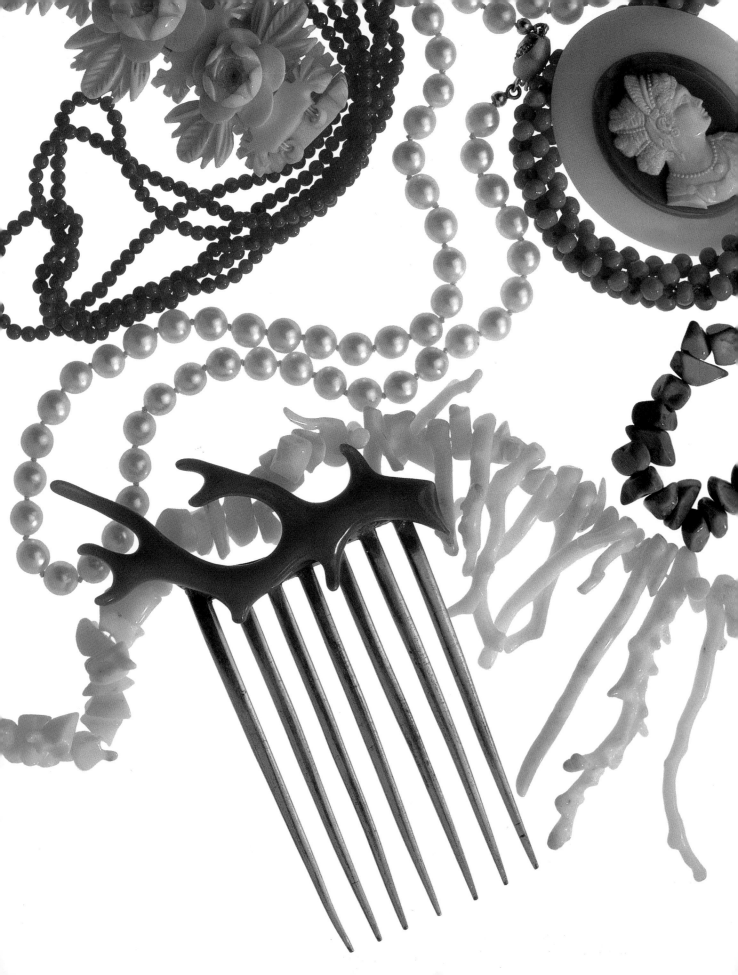

That special finishing touch

JEWELLERY COLOURS

Basically, jewellery is nothing more than another accessory. Each piece has its own colours – just like a scarf, a belt or a pair of shoes. But – as far as colour is concerned – who will part with a much-loved ring or necklace just because it doesn't fit into her charts? No-one; jewellery is personal and sentimental.

Jewellery is a personal choice

Almost every woman possesses some jewellery – maybe just wedding ring, a little heart necklace or sometimes something expensive and precious. She may, of course, leave expensive items in the safe and wear paste copies on special occasions, or she may wear a lot of jewellery every day. Certainly, over a period of time, a woman amasses a very personal, sentimental collection – a wooden bangle, a silver ring bought on holiday or a glass stone clip from a boutique, plus earrings that once she just had to buy. And don't forget family treasures – a locket inherited from a grandmother, a mother's pearl necklace or a charm bracelet which has been added to over the years.

There will be presents received from time to time – from relatives, friends and ex-friends – and those items she loved so much she bought them for herself. A modern woman has no hesitation in ignoring tradition and buying jewellery for herself if she knows it will look terrific.

So let's try to consider jewellery as an accessory – whether fashion jewellery or genuine stones – exactly like a belt, a bag or a stunning pair of shoes. Jewellery tells people who we are; it styles our clothes in a particular manner (classical, elegant, fashionable or outrageous) and highlights our own individuality.

And jewellery is personal. It is part of us, our background and our family, part of our past romances and fond memories. We may throw away an old pullover or a worn-out coat but who would discard a ring (even with two missing stones) when its style no longer fits in with our lives? For this reason it is difficult to be firm in fitting jewellery into the colour type rules. Certainly, you are not going to get rid of a precious piece simply because it does not fit in with your colour chart. On the other hand you may discover your new awareness of colours means you now wear only certain pieces. Maybe because they incorporate your colours and so you instinctively wear them, perhaps daily. Other pieces you leave in the box. Even so, it is a good idea to check whether your favoured items fit into your colour chart.

But as with the colour white, gold – particularly – has several different colour variations. Pure gold, for example, is a powerful, sunny yellow, but it is too soft for jewellery. Jewellery made of pure gold would quickly bend and wear out so it is mixed with other hard metals. These metals change the colour of the gold, producing distinctly 'cool' and 'warm' tones.

Silver has a cool effect: gold can be warm or cool depending on its mixture of metals.

Normal yellow gold is mixed with silver and copper and always has a warm appearance. Red gold has a high percentage of copper and can, depending on the tone, be warm as well as cool, while light red gold contains silver (as well as copper). The silver gives light red gold a delicate, cool shimmer. White gold is made of gold that has been mixed with platinum and nickel – a cool effect. When gold is mixed with steel it has a cool blue shine; mixed with cadmium and silver, it is a greenish gold. Old Victorian jewellery usually has a soft red gold shimmer – red gold was very popular at the time – and its soft, gentle appeal is much valued as an alternative to the brilliance of modern jewellery. Jewellery from Germany's Biedermeier period of the early to mid-19th century, however beautiful, often only has a layer of yellow gold plate, while items from the Art Nouveau and Art Deco periods are mostly made of white gold or silver. It's obvious; once you take your time to really look at gold there is a wide range of different gold 'colours' available.

At the less expensive end of the jewellery market, there is little gold in gold-plate jewellery, where a thin layer is rolled into another metal, usually steel. In the case of all imitation gold jewellery the only 'gold' remaining is the colour but even here the colours can be varied depending on whether the mixture is copper with tin (brass), copper with zinc (bronze) or whether the imitation gold has been made with artificial materials.

Silver jewellery has always been popular and suits large, dramatic pieces. It reminds us of the coolness of the moon's rays and a good piece shows off this precious metal to its best effect (especially graceful– and with a cold tone – is artificially blackened silver). And finally we have platinum – an extremely valuable and precious metal which, if we are not careful, can sometimes be taken for silver.

Large jewellery and fine, delicate jewellery – select the right one for your type.

As far as precious and semi-precious stones are concerned, jewellery with diamonds, crystal and paste are cool – with no colour to detract the eye it is the cold flash of the stones that fascinate. Coloured stones can be soft and delicate, fiery and glowing, and warm or cold. If you are undecided whether or not a piece complements your type, place the stone against your colour chart. See whether it harmonises with the colours and appears alive. Or do the colours dominate the stone, rendering it invisible?

As we have said, we know you will always treasure your own, personal jewellery collection –

whatever the result of the colour test. However, next time you pay a visit to the jeweller's shop, you will know what suits you and will be able to choose a piece which is not only beautiful and valuable, but also attractive ... for you.

Every precious stone, including a colourless diamond, has a unique character.

So why not do it? Sort out your fashion jewellery – it shouldn't be too difficult. That African wooden bangle in marvellous natural colours is perfect for the Autumn woman, but does not suit you now you know you are a Winter type who looks better in diamonds (even if imitation). You always knew that the bangle would never make you look attractive. And what about those May green plastic earrings which are perfect for a Spring type, but you are Summer! Or those grey plastic pearls which you know are not 'you'; try swopping them for another colour.

Jewellery for the Spring type

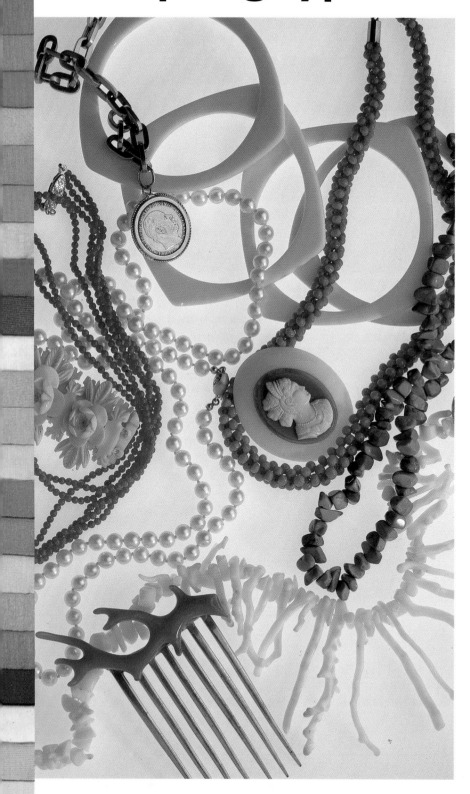

'Delicate and fine' is the ideal jewellery for the Spring woman; large, bold pieces look crude. You can, however, wear powerful colours – turquoise, rich topaz, blue sapphire or yellow amber – all colours that are found on your colour chart. Many warm jewellery colours suit Spring people including natural coral and, of course, warm ivory-coloured items. If you like wearing pearls remember that cream-white or yellow suit you best and that yellow gold or red gold jewellery complement you perfectly (never white gold or silver).

Jewellery for the Summer type

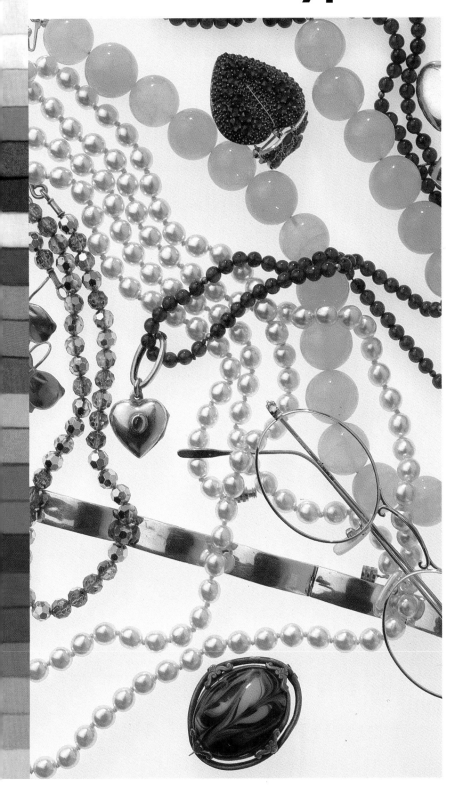

Summer women tend to look good in old, matt rather than shiny jewellery; as far as colours are concerned Summer women should opt for cool and soft colours. Stones such as rubies or garnet are perfect – bright but not gaudy. Other stones suitable for the Summer woman are milky, blue opals, soft blue aquamarine and green jade (bluish rather than green), as well as grey-blue or grey-green agate. Naturally diamonds are also suitable for the Summer type! And pearls in grey and rose. In the case of gold, white or cool red gold should be considered – yellow gold does not suit the Summer type. And silver is excellent.

Jewellery for the Autumn type

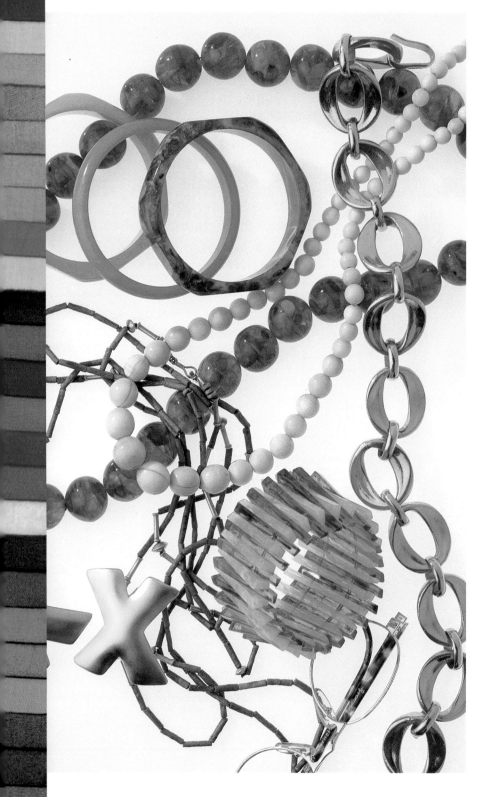

Autumn women prefer the natural look. Bangles made of wood and plastic in the colour of yellow ivory, necklaces of amber or bone-coloured material, leather and feather jewellery, everything that looks as natural as autumn colours. Without over-doing it, the Autumn type can also wear large jewellery but take care not to choose shiny, gleaming pieces as these dominate your natural soft colours. Richly coloured stones are stunning – strong red coral, yellow green jade, golden yellow topaz, warm agate, and warm, creamy pearls. Gold can also be worn – not white gold – as can copper and bronze, but silver is unsuitable.

Jewellery for the Winter type

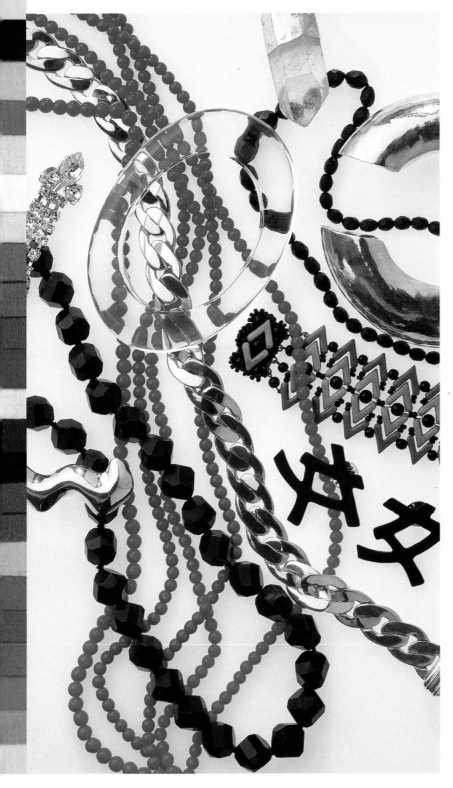

The more extravagant the better for Winter women. These women look particularly good in diamonds, crystal and paste, and large, sparkling pieces – hoops and large plastic earrings – look terrific because they emphasise the contrast of Winter's dramatic colouring. Discreet can be boring. Winter types can carry powerful colours – sultry onyx or black jet, wine red rubies, deep green emerald (and imitation items of similar richness). If Winter women wear pearls, they should choose several strings of cool white, grey or black pearls and Winter's metals are platinum, white gold, silver; never yellow gold.

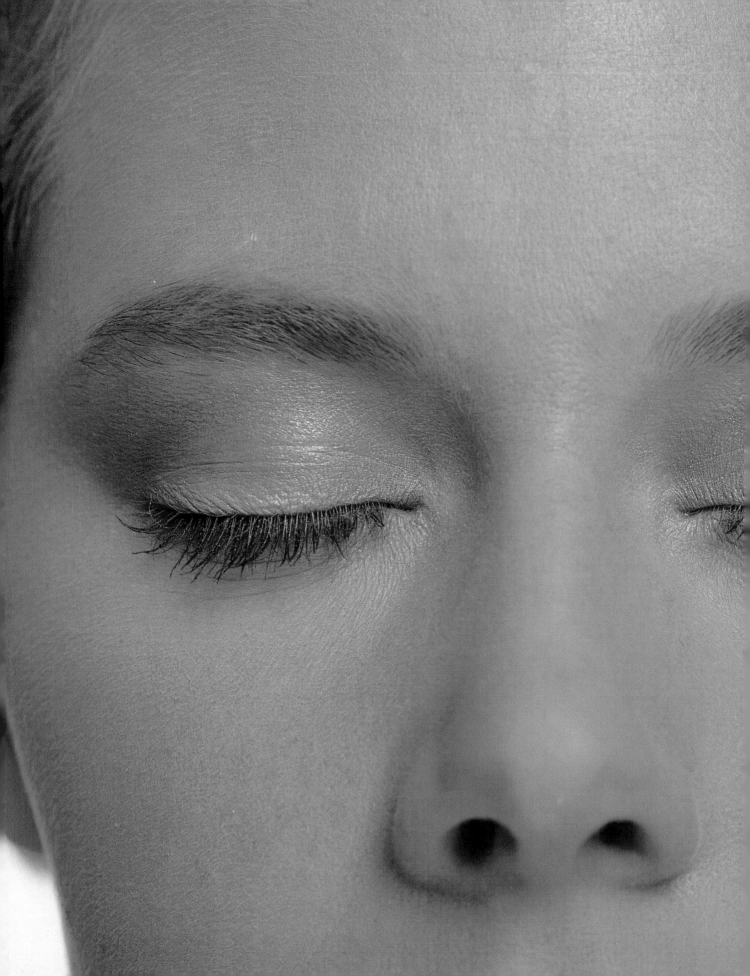

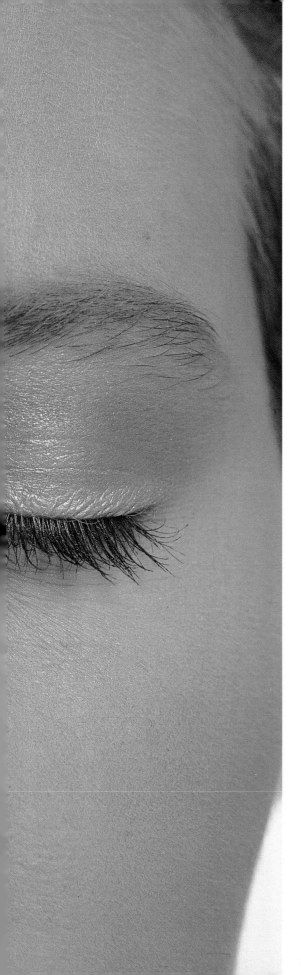

COSMETIC COLOURS

Naturally, the right make-up colours are crucial: cool, clear colours for Summer and Winter women; warm for the Spring and Autumn types. Why? Because what is right for clothes is even more important for the face – the complexion, eyes and hair colours. Keeping to your colour type ensures a finished, polished effect.

Prettier with the right make-up

Naturally, there are women who have even, faultless and finely-pored skin who are beautiful without cosmetics – natural beauties who look well groomed and made-up with only a touch of lipstick. However, most of us need a little help to look good and we get this from make-up which is applied carefully, fashionably and attractively.

The correct foundation is vital. Choose one that is lighter rather than darker than your natural skin colour.

This is not meant to be an in-depth course in make-up; we only want to suggest a few basic rules, important for every colour type.

The most difficult choice to make is foundation. However, as you now know your colour type, you will find this a lot easier. Cosmetic companies usually have four to six different foundation colours in their ranges. The lightest and the darkest are of little use to most women – they are too fashionable or too extreme. Let the sales assistant show you all the others and take a good, long look ... which ones have a yellow 'warm' tone (Spring and Autumn types) and which a rosy grey 'cool' tone (Summer and Winter)? Compare the colours against each other directly. Take the foundation to a window and look at it in daylight. Don't feel intimidated.

The colour of the foundation should match your own complexion – or as near as possible – so that both colours blend into each other easily. And if undecided – always choose a lighter rather than a darker colour! If the foundation is too dark everyone will see a line where it stops, it highlights wrinkles and often looks artificial. And remember – don't test the foundation on the back of the hand or on the inside of the wrist. Make-up artists always advise trying out foundation on your forehead – it has a truer colour and you are less likely to make an expensive mistake.

Never buy a new foundation just after a summer or skiing holiday. Your skin should then look good enough to do without make-up and it is practically impossible to match foundation to natural sun-tanned tones.

How to apply foundation? Remember, a light touch is best if you want to see the face, not the make-up.

Just a word about the consistency of foundation: very liquid foundations have a natural, transparent sheen, but do not cover imperfections such as red veins, while the thicker, cream-style foundations do a good cover-up job but need special care. If they are applied with a heavy hand you will feel and look tacky and uncomfortable.

Foundation must be applied very evenly and lightly, preferably with a small sponge.

If you have minor imperfections, first use a matching skin concealer to disguise these. Then for a light, transparent effect, carefully and evenly apply the liquid foundation directly to the skin using either your (clean) fingertips or a small, slightly damp make-up sponge. Never rub the colour in. Then very lightly powder the foundation to 'set' it. This is your base – perfect whether you now require a simple, minimal make-up or a more time-consuming, glamorous evening look.

Even eyeshadow, lipstick and blusher should be chosen from your colour range.

As with clothes, accessories and jewellery, lipstick, blusher and eyeshadow should harmonise with your colour chart. Have a look at the many cosmetics companies' samples on display within stores and shops – you will find both cool and dramatic colours as well as earthy and warm themes. And remember that cosmetic manufacturers often choose a colour palette for a season – like fashion designers. Maybe Company X has only autumn or copper colours one year which, as a Summer type, you know don't suit you. Choose another company for a while; one which has the cool, blue tones you now know you need.

Once you know your colour chart well you will instinctively know which are the right make-up colours for you. As a general rule, colours which suit you in a blouse or shirt should also look terrific on your face or eyes (in a more subdued version, of course).

Naturally, when choosing eyeshadow it is not necessary to try out every colour you see; just choose a few that harmonise with your eyes. On the following pages you will find hints as to which colours these are (and which lipstick and blushers suit you best).

Nail varnish and lipstick should suit your type, but do not need to match.

Perhaps you have seen a nail varnish that looks good on someone else, but on you it looks disappointing? Something went wrong. Certainly your nails were noticeable but you felt uncomfortable. Maybe your hands looked rougher and your nails looked as though they did not belong to you!

The prettiest warm coral red looks ordinary if applied to nails on hands with a cool blue undertone to the skin, and lively rose pink can look vulgar on a hand with warm yellow skin tones. A face can be powdered (making the wrong foundation look better), but if hand colours clash the mistake is obvious.

Matching your lipstick and nail varnish is a long outdated concept. Ignore it.

Obviously lipstick and blusher should harmonise because they are positioned near to each other, but it is enough if your nail varnish is of the same 'warmth' or 'coolness' as your lipstick colour. Their tones should co-ordinate, but whether one is lighter or darker than the other really doesn't matter any more – they will go well with each other.

The Spring type: delicate and natural

The worst make-up for the Spring type is a strong and dramatic one. Under no circumstances should Spring types look plastered with make-up – their special radiance depends entirely on their delicate, transparent complexion which requires only a gentle emphasis to look stunning. This means using a 'warm' liquid foundation which matches her skin; never a compact, thick foundation. An apricot or peach blusher is perfect, best swept over a large area of the face to eliminate any hard contrasts, and a warm, rosy lipstick colour completes the Spring make-up. If a Spring woman wishes to wear a powerful red lipstick – which can look terrific – she should remember to look for a warm coral or lobster red, never a bluish red, such as ruby or fuchsia. Incidentally, if wearing this strong, powerful red, always choose a glossy lipstick (not one with a matt, powder cover); Spring types are the only women who look good with lips and eyes made up to roughly the same strength. On other women it can appear boring or obtrusive, but on them it looks discreet and natural. When it comes to eye make-up the Spring woman would do best to choose milky, soft colours to give a warm, natural effect (see page 92). Coloured mascara is perfect. Its hint of colour allows the Spring woman to fully experiment with colour without running the risk of looking gaudy.

The Spring woman's fresh, delicate colouring must not be covered or altered with make-up. By using the correct warm and light tones she will look attractive and natural, not painted. Light milky tones are good for Spring's eyes with a peach red for blusher and lipstick.

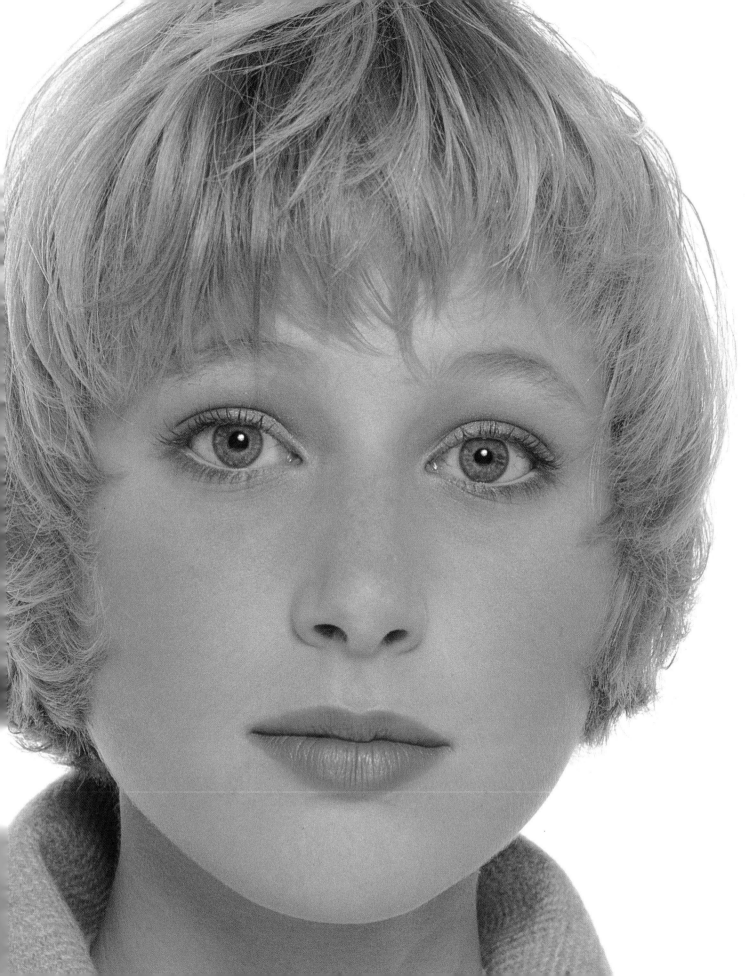

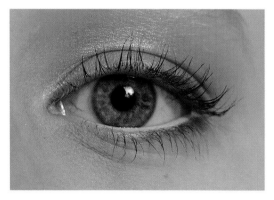

Photo left: a salmon shadow with nougat brown towards the outer edge is complimented by dark brown mascara and white kajal.
Photo below: blue eyes are accentuated by pastel green eyeshadow, green mascara and white kajal (a brown shadow, too, looks good with blue eyes).

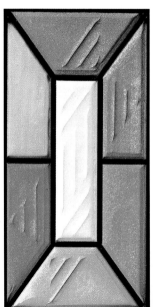

Always remember – make-up in its packaging looks more intense than on the skin. Shown, left, is a typical Spring palette with photographs showing how these colours look when applied. Especially pretty combinations are nougat brown, linden green and a soft white; light lilac, delicate turquoise and ochre; delicate rose, linden green and nougat brown, or ochre, light lilac and, again, nougat brown. When mixing eye colours remember to apply the darkest colour first, mixing this with the lighter ones.

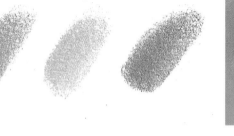

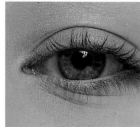

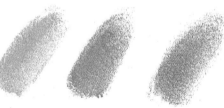

Photo right: a very natural-looking lipstick colour. Lightly outline the lips with a delicate rose-brown pencil before filling in.
Photo below: clear, rose-brown lip colours always suit the Spring woman.

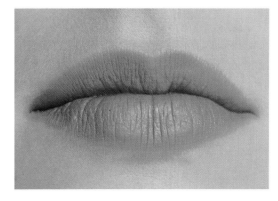

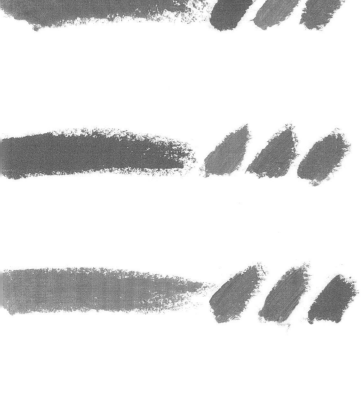

Spring women look good with either a very delicate, glossy lip colour or a stronger, more defined lipstick but the more natural the lips, the prettier they are. Soft, gentle oranges are attractive as are peach and light, earthy rose-browns (if not too dull); for a change, a full brilliant lobster red looks stunning.
Shown, right, are Spring's preferred lipstick colours while the colour samples, left, show four typical colours (the broad colour strip harmonises with the eyeshadows opposite).

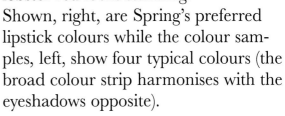

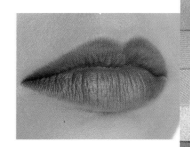

The Summer type: cool and softly smokey

Summer women are lucky – they can indulge themselves with colours, (while always remembering these should be 'cool'), as their stronger skin tones can carry the more intense cosmetic colours. A deep, rich lipstick or a cool, shimmering eyeshadow make a flattering contrast to the warm skin tone and reserved ash blonde or ash brown hair colours. Summer women too, have more choice – do they want to look natural or sporty (with a light foundation and a slick of lipstick?), or more elegant with a full, powdered make-up and defined, fully painted lips? And what of the so-called French make-up – a little blusher, some powder and a strong dramat-ic red mouth? The Summer woman can have it all. Naturally, the French make-up's blusher should be in the same cool colour spectrum as the lipstick and must never overpower it – no-one wants to look 'painted'. Other Summer women may choose to emphasise their eyes instead of their lips and with their grey-blue or grey-brown eyes they have a whole palette of colours from which to choose. The best cool colours for Summer types are shown on page 96, and include a smokey brown instead of nougat brown and a sharp, fluorescent yellow instead of rich, egg-yolk yellow. However, don't be timid. If you wish to mix a favourite, 'warm' colour with your chart's cooler shades, it won't hurt. Have a bit of fun. Just remember it is important that the colours closest to your coloured iris are taken from the correct colour palette.

A brilliant bluish red mouth with a perfectly drawn outline livens up a Summer face and acts as an important accent. But to balance this the blusher should be restrained, with soft, refined eyes. All cool make-up colours are ideal for the Summer woman.

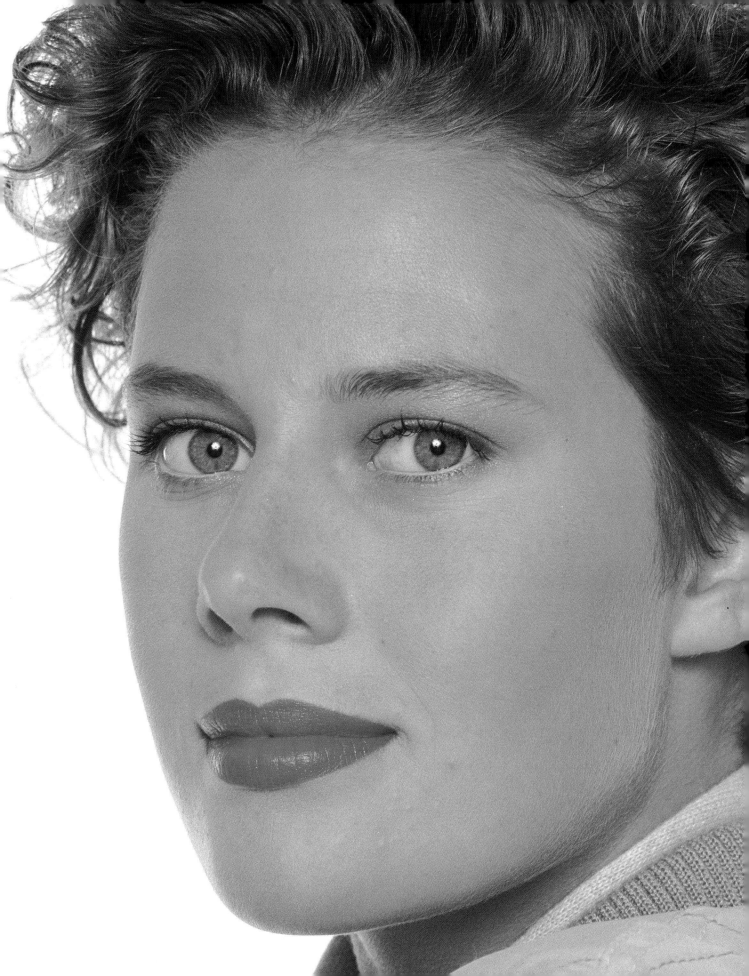

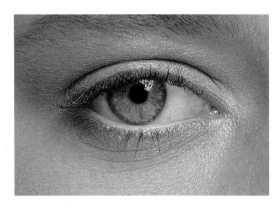

A playground of colours for the Summer type. Photo, left: pastel green lids, dark violet on the lower lid, lighter on the arch of the brows. Photo below: rose to blue-violet over the fold of the eyelid and in the corner of the eye, silver white highlighter on the lid. On the lower lid a little colour with white kajal.

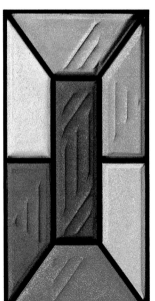

A Summer's make-up colours are cool but full of colour. Shown, left, is a typical Summer palette; the photographs show the same colours after application. Should the lid make-up dominate, dust with light face powder. Grey, from silver to anthracite, and grey-brown are the ideal eyeshadow colours for Summer women who want subtlety: for a more dramatic effect Summer types can combine violet, blue and green; green, pale yellow and pink; rose, violet and blue, or light yellow, blue and silver white.

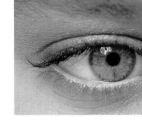

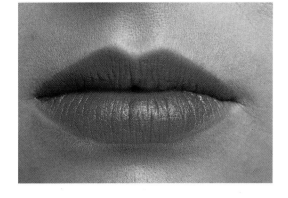

Fully painted lips with an accurate, defined outline are an important focal point. Photo right: a light bluish melon colour suits the Summer woman just as well as the full bluish red lip tones.
Photo below: a soft, almost mauve, rose is equally complementary to the Summer type.

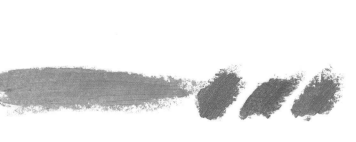

There is a wide, stunning range of light to dark lipstick colours available to the Summer woman. 'Baby rose' is not ideal; choose a more graceful, reserved old rose or a lively pink. The middle or dark colours tend towards blue – fuchsias and azalea shades – while the clearest red tends towards purple. Many reserved, unobtrusive violet variations can be worn well by the Summer woman as can the gentle melon reds or delicate mallows. Shown right, are four suitable lipsticks; shown left, are four colour samples.

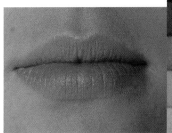

The Autumn type: warm and radiant

Those Autumn women with dark complexions and deep, richly coloured eyes look terrific without make-up. But for those types with pale skin and lightly-coloured hair a touch of make-up is necessary to enhance their natural characteristics. And Autumn types have the choice of a natural, tone-on-tone make-up or of fashionably experimenting with the latest colours. Both can look stunningly attractive. The light skinned Autumn woman should choose a clear, thin liquid foundation – a wisp is enough to give colour to the face and powder is often not required. Most Autumn types instinctively choose earthy, natural colours. But soft brown lips with soft brown eyeshadows can look boring. Autumn women should experiment – try out all the many different 'warm' gold colours while not forgetting some 'cool' colours. For example, a tomato red or gold-effect, warm lipstick looks exciting when used by the Autumn woman, while a blackberry tending towards aubergine can look unbelievably attractive (colours the Autumn woman should avoid include the light mother-of-pearl, icy lilac or a cold pink rose – much too cold). The same rule applies for eyeshadow: soft nougat and copper look natural and elegant, but a shimmer of tile green or warm lilac can look stunningly different. Autumn women can make up their eyes strongly and dramatically but if they wish to avoid looking flashy they should then tone down their lipstick. And vice versa: an emphasised mouth demands a gentler approach to the eyes.

Autumn types have the choice between making up naturally in the soft brown tones of their colour range, or using a more obvious, extravagant make-up. Always attractive, however, are intensified colours around the edge of the eye lashes with a natural glossy mouth.

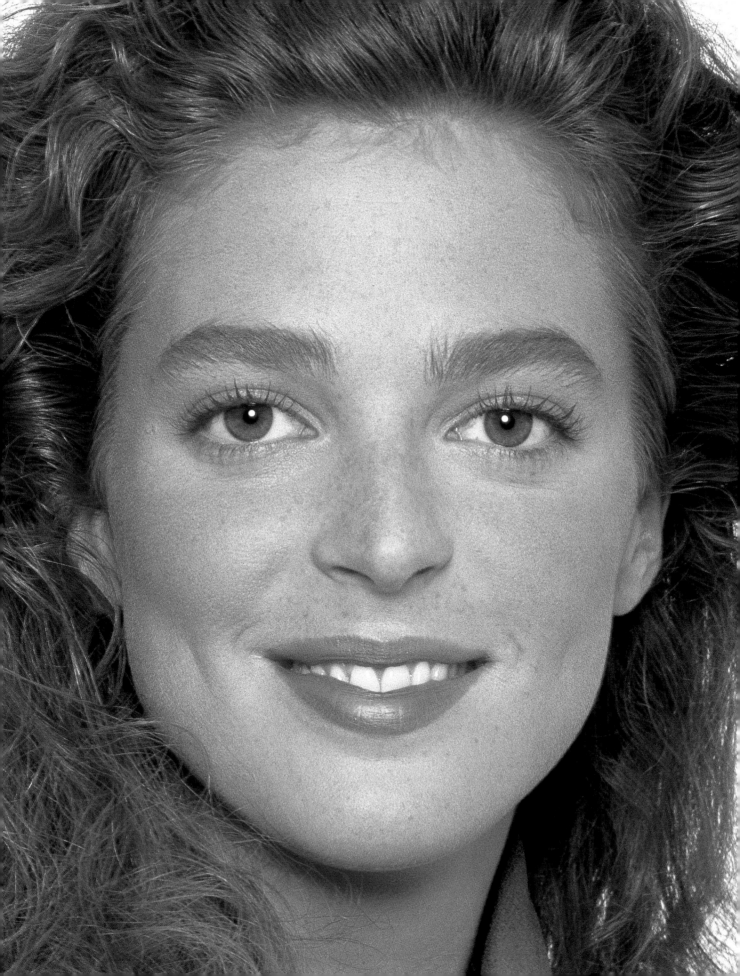

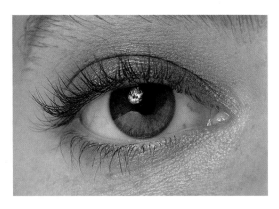

Photo, left: for a change from brown-on-brown, these dark eyes are highlighted with a taffeta green on the lids and in the socket, with light brown on the browbone, and salmon on the lower lid.

Photo below: an aubergine shadow on the eyelid with night blue at the lash edge and a light kajal on the lower lid.

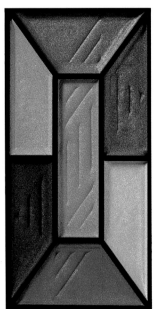

Autumn types can use rich, deep colours. They have dark eyes which are complemented by similarly strong eyeshadows. But alongside all the usual copper and brown tones, don't forget Autumn women look good in dark aubergine, lavender or a light leaf green with salmon, peach or sun yellow for lighter accentuating touches.

Shown left, is Autumn's colour palette: right, the same colours as they look when applied. Particularly pretty are combinations of lavender, aubergine and copper; leaf green, peach and salmon; aubergine, peach and sun yellow, or lavender, leaf green and peach. A special tip: brush a light colour over the lower-lid dark colours.

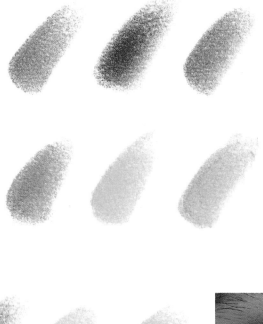

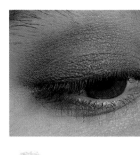

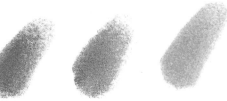

Matt or glossy lips are suitable for the Autumn woman.
Photo right: a glossy, gold-coloured lipstick is carefully and generously applied.
Photo below: a burgundy lipstick is softened to a gentle, raspberry colour when lightly powdered.

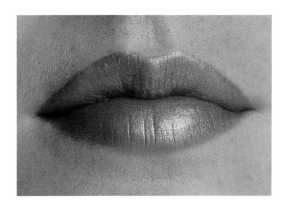

But what happens when you prefer a brown or orange lipstick? Or a really bright red and a shimmering copper tone? As an Autumn woman you can choose between all these colours. For example, a tomato red suits you well as does a full salmon red, a shimmering copper and – unusual and very dramatic – a dark bluish-blackberry red. Shown, right, are the lipsticks and left, colour samples of four typical lipstick colours for the Autumn woman. The widely drawn strip of colour goes especially well with those eye shadow combinations on the opposite page. Incidentally, it is worth noting that only Autumn women can wear a true orange!

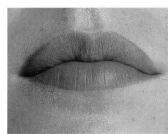

The Winter type: Thriving on contrasts

A Winter face is marked by strong colour contrasts between skin and hair, and between the iris and the whites of the eyes. Of course, there are exceptions to every rule but when it comes to make-up the following applies to every Winter type – too much colour is very ordinary. The Winter woman needs only a few, strong colours. As a base, Winter's normal, light complexion requires an equally light foundation (even if there is an olive undertone) and, normally, little blusher is needed. Where it is used, it should have the same colour tone as the lipstick and be evenly spread. A strong lipstick colour is advised, balanced with a subtle, clear eye make-up in a light-dark contrast. If, however, she chooses only the slightest trace of lip gloss the Winter woman can dramatically emphasise her hypnotic eyes with a dark khol, painting her eyelids with deep, dark colours. For example, the Winter woman is perfect for 60's make-up – rose-white lips with black, starkly outlined eyes. And she is the only one of the four types to benefit from defining her eyes with a blue-red kajal without the red making her look as if she has been crying! But a word of warning: Winter types with an olive-coloured complexion can mistakenly believe themselves to be Autumn women and make up accordingly. While a few may find that Autumn's colour palette will suit them, most Winter women will look yellowish and unattractive. Her preferred, cool colours make her look good – whether close-up or from a distance!

Winter women need only a few, strong make-up colours: either accentuating their lips with a clear red or using dramatic, expressive eye colours. But not both together; this has an over-done effect. Most Winter types do not need much blusher.

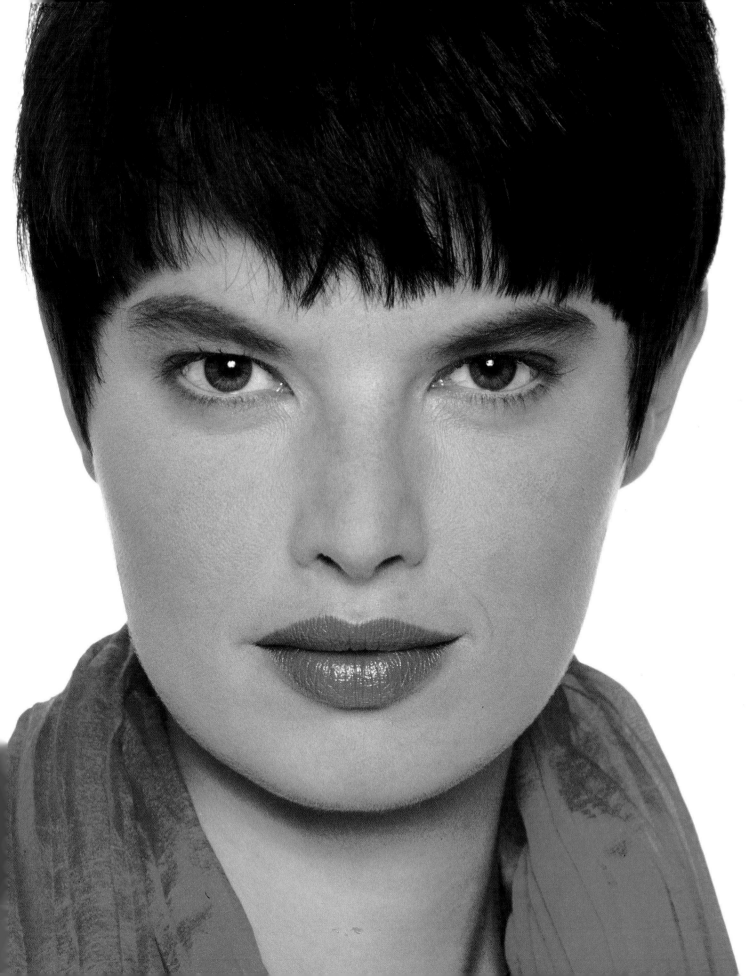

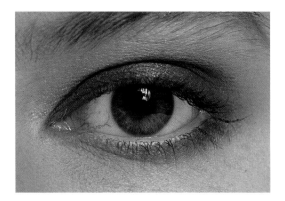

Photo, left: the eye is totally framed in a single petrol green, a style in which winter types always look good. Photo, below: a very discreet, refined and quite a different approach - anthracite from the brow to the eyelid folds, with a touch of pink on the lids.

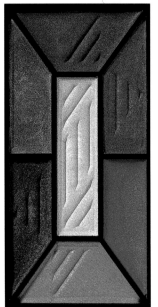

The Winter woman can experiment with rich, dark colours – deep, intense mauve; smokey brown; anthracite; dark blue and dark green – but not all at the same time! What is important is the light-dark contrast, not the number of colours used. Shown, left, is Winter's typical colour palette: shown, right, are the same colours when applied. Should the Winter woman wish to mix the dif-ferent colours the best are smoke brown, rose and anthracite; mauve, night blue and a tiny trace of pink (more to lighten than as a basic colour); dark green, night blue and rose to lighten, or an almost tone-on-tone pink, mauve and rose applied sparingly.

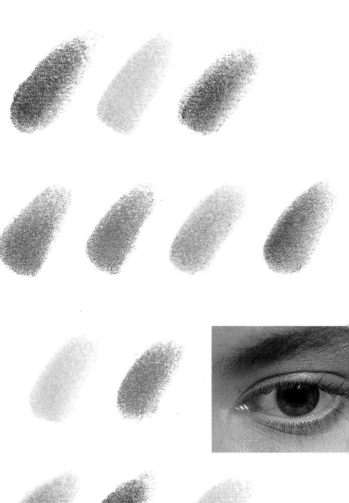

Simple, glossy lips work well when the eyes are dramatically made up. A quite different effect can be created by outlining with a darker lip liner and filling with colour. Photo, right: a pink-coloured lip gloss (sometimes a coat of colourless lip gloss looks pretty). Photo, below: a brilliant, deep winter red.

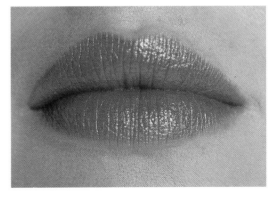

For the Winter woman clear and definite bluish reds are the best lipstick colours. This is not a time for subtlety! And what may look gaudy on other women suits her very well indeed. She can wear a very icy pink, but also Picasso red, brilliant cyclamen and a strong cherry red. Shown, right: the four Winter lipsticks and, left: Winter's colour samples. The widely drawn strip of colour is best suited to the eyelid shadow combinations on the left. Another tip: Winter women should always outline their lips after applying lipstick to give a stronger appearance.

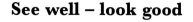

See well – look good

COLOURS
FOR GLASSES

As any woman who has to wear glasses knows, not only do they change her appearance, but they can alter the over-all view of herself.

Ultimately, glasses cannot be missed. They are positioned in the middle of the face and the best thing to do is to turn them into an attractive accessory. To work with them, not against them. Pay attention to their shape and colour, and whether or not their shape suits you.

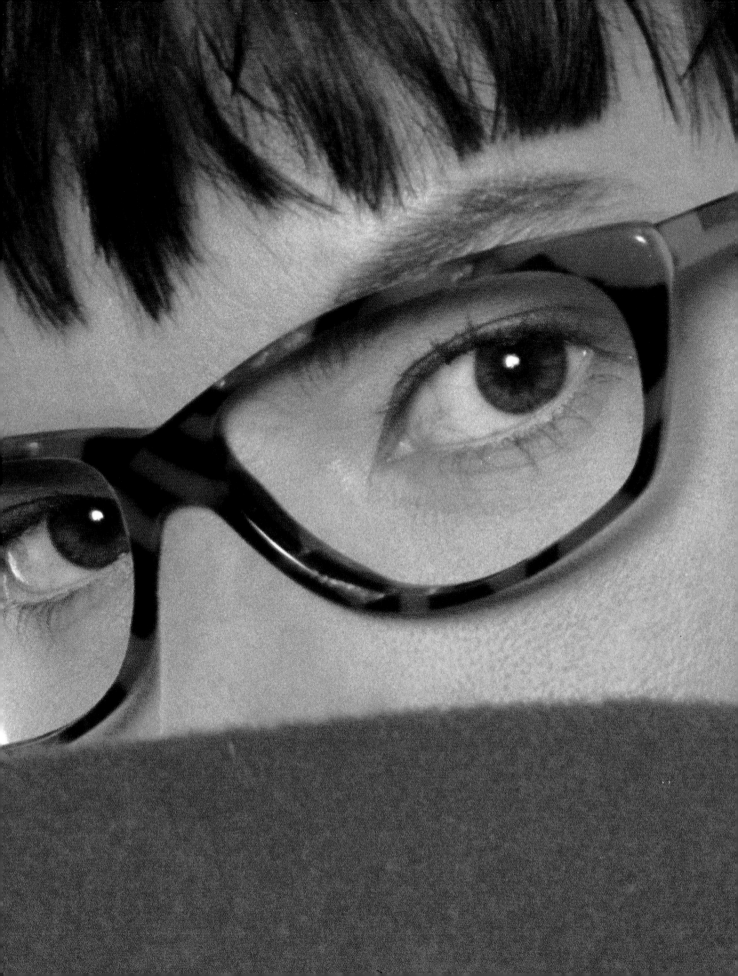

Glasses – a necessary accessory

Do you have to wear glasses all the time, or only occasionally? Even if you only need them from time to time, it is important that you choose them in the same way as you choose your make-up colours and hair styles. You may not be able to see them, but they are highly visible to others! They take up a dominant position on your face and have a decisive effect on your whole appearance.

At best, wearing glasses can actually improve a woman's appearance! Do you recall times when you have been speaking with a woman who has been wearing glasses who has then taken them off for cleaning and you have found yourself thinking, 'But she doesn't look nearly as good without her glasses!' If the colour and shape of the chosen glasses harmonise with the skin tone, hair colour and shape of a woman's face, they will suit not only her appearance but also her personality.

The ideal glasses: fashionable, and a natural part of you.

Choosing glasses is a major purchasing decision. You are not only spending a fair amount of money, but you are making a decision which can radically change your appearance. Whether for the better or not is up to you. If you make a colour mistake when buying a lipstick or blouse, it is irritating but not a major problem. If you make a mistake with your glasses, however, it is far more serious. Take your time to assess which colour is best for you and which is the right shape. Treat them as a part of yourself, your wardrobe and your lifestyle.

Today, you can buy glasses frames in any and every colour. When choosing, take your colour chart with you just as you might when buying cosmetics and clothes. If a colour is right for you in a lipstick or a shirt, then it is probably right for your frames.

But a note of caution: the colour intensity of the frames can still be too strong or too weak. If you have a delicate face choosing a pair of glasses with frames from the darker end of your colour chart may be too strong (even if it suits you well as a shirt or a scarf). For example, maybe you have a dark complexion? If so, you should avoid choosing light, almost transparent tones on your chart for your frames. For such an important decision, take you time and try as many coloured pairs as you can.

A tip: patterned frames might be easier for you. Particularly fashionable and optically interesting, these have a softer effect than single-colour frames because the shape is 'broken-up' by the pattern.

Metal or plastic? Single colour or with a pattern? It all depends on the colour.

Frames can be speckled, 'marbled', imitation tortoiseshell or with a general, specially designed pattern. The same pair of patterned glasses can look different, depending on the colour of the clothing worn. For example, a blue-grey pair of glasses can look good with blue, grey or other related colours and may take on a slightly different hue with each colour. What's more, the materials used affect the colour decision – metal, plastic, or combined? (Suggestions as to which glasses go well with which colour type can be found from pp. 110.)

If you choose, say, metal frames over coloured plastic ones, then because your glasses are simply just another piece of jewellery, make sure the rest of your jewellery co-ordinates. The cool types – Summer and Winter – might do well to choose silver, or blackened-silver frames, and some Summer women could also wear cool, red gold frames (but never yellow gold which are more suitable for Spring and Autumn types!). These women also suit engraved, matt metal frames which have an 'antique' appearance, particularly the delicate Spring women on whom a shiny frame would look out-of-place.

If you prefer 'real' material to metal, plastic and imitations, buffalo horn frames are now available (instead of the now protected tortoiseshell). Clearly, horn is ideal for the Autumn woman and her natural, earthy colour options, but it is also suitable for women with allergies to either metal or plastic. Everyone suffering from the irritating nickel allergy should be aware that all metal frames contain some nickel.

Another tip: coloured lenses are available for women who have to wear glasses at all times throughout the day. The right lens colour can emphasise your choice of frame and act as a true accessory. But you must never choose coloured lenses for reading glasses. These are worn only occasionally and it is essential that as much light as possible passes through the lens. The glass must be clear and sharp.

When glasses are worn all day and every day, have some fun and choose tinted glasses for maximum personal impact! If the colour is carefully chosen and not too strong, they will not impair your vision. You will not be looking at a green, blue or rose-coloured world; the difference is minimal and barely noticeable. However, be guided by your optician; he knows the colour strength should not be more than twelve per cent. A higher percentage of colour makes the eyes light-sensitive – like wearing sunglasses all the time.

Looking at the world through rose-tinted glasses? Possible – and flattering.

Glass lenses are available only in grey, brown and rose colours; plastic lenses, however, are available in a wide choice of colours – from blue, green and turquoise through violet, rose and orange to brown and grey, and in all colour intensities. Let the optician guide you; he will explain the many options. Place the glass lenses under your chosen frame and take a long look at yourself in the mirror. You now know your best colours – Summer and Winter women should go for cool-coloured glass lenses, a bluish rose, grey or turquoise green colour, or even a light reddish violet. Spring and Autumn types look better with warm lenses – say, a light yellow or soft orange yellow, with beige or brown. Rimless glasses look very effective with coloured lenses as do those glasses with just a single bar at the top. Normal clear glass lenses can be featureless; tinted lenses add character and individuality.

Glasses for the Spring type

Frames in (from the top) soft tiger stripes, transparent salmon rose, lobster red and light brown and beige – four styles for the Spring woman. She could also try soft blue, delicate yellow, perhaps ivory-coloured or a very light buffalo horn – all light colours which will harmonise with her skin, hair and make-up colours. What frames should the Spring woman never wear? Black, blue, green, bluish red and similarly strong colours. And metal? The Spring woman should choose a matt yellow gold.

How to choose the right frame? Simple – the only way is to try them out, again and again. A general rule is that the shape of the glasses should not echo the shape of the face, but work against it. So, no square frames for angular faces, no round frames for round faces, no pearl-drop shapes for long faces (choose a square shape instead).

Glasses for the Summer type

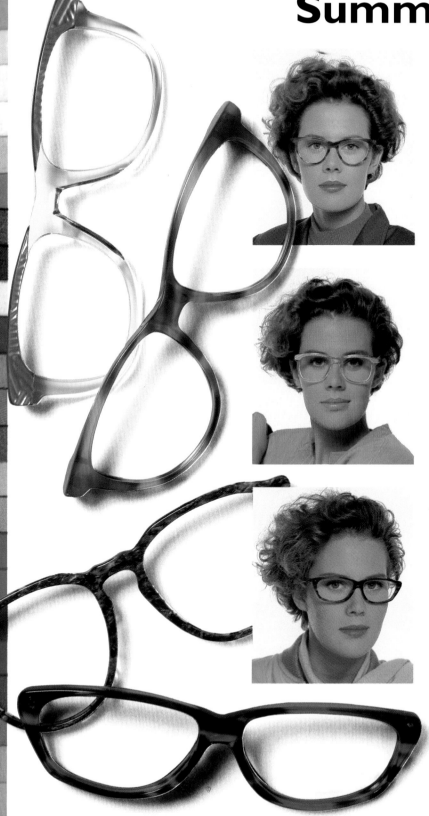

The Summer woman cannot go wrong with the silver grey transparent frames (top) – they are ideal for her cool complexion and ashy hair tone. The shaded, patterned amethyst pair harmonise with the many colours in her chart, but she could probably also carry the more outrageous green marbled and dark red and black frames – ideal for a second pair of glasses. Generally speaking, the Summer woman can choose from most cool, subdued colours and she also looks good in silver or cool red gold metal frames.

Glasses for the Autumn type

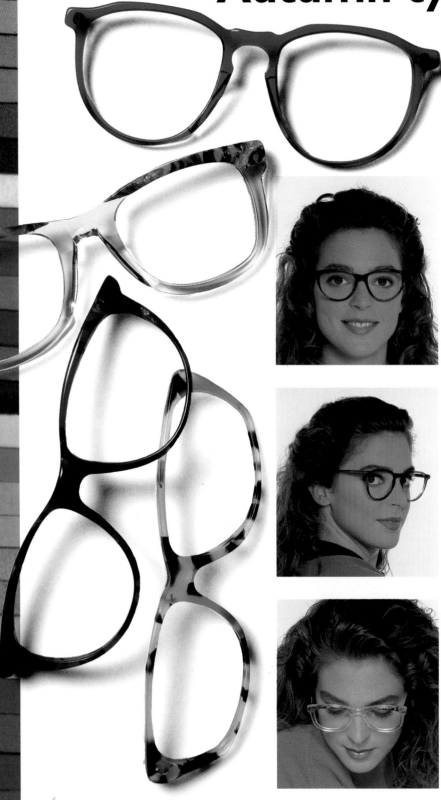

Suitable for Autumn types are warm, full frames and only those with a pale skin should choose transparent or light patterns. Autumn types should avoid all cool colours. Examples of frames in powerful colours are the blue-red frames (top), and the green and red patterned ones (second from bottom). Also suitable for the Autumn woman are warm brown, rust and a clear jade green. A wonderfully light effect is offered by transparent frames with a coloured upper part (second from top) and the dramatic yellow and brown tiger stripe (bottom). Light, pretty Autumn colours would also be amber, light red or salmon, and frames made of horn and those in yellow gold or copper tones suit her equally well.

Glasses for the Winter type

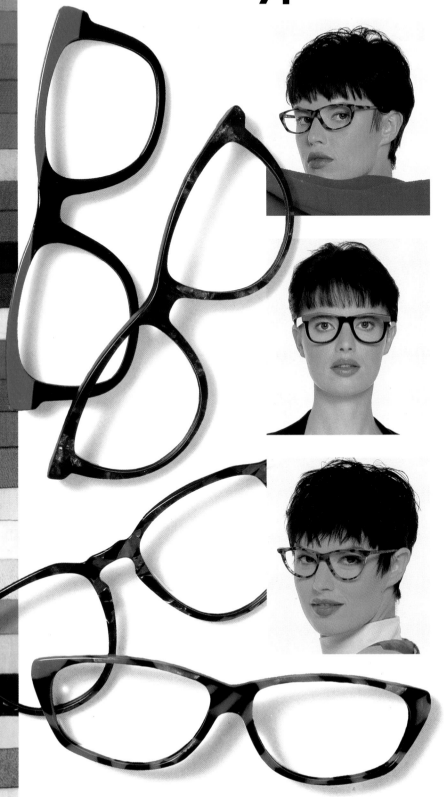

Dark, opaque frames in full, cool tones are ideal for Winter types. Blue and black frames (top) look dramatic and stunning, while the anthracite frames with silver marbling are softer. More lively options for the Winter woman are frames that highlight her colour contrasts – try red and black patterned frames (bottom) or cool green, lilac and black frames. And what to choose for a second pair? Try the other colours in Winter's chart – fuchsia red, ruby red or pine green. And if metal is preferred, try silver or black-ened-silver.

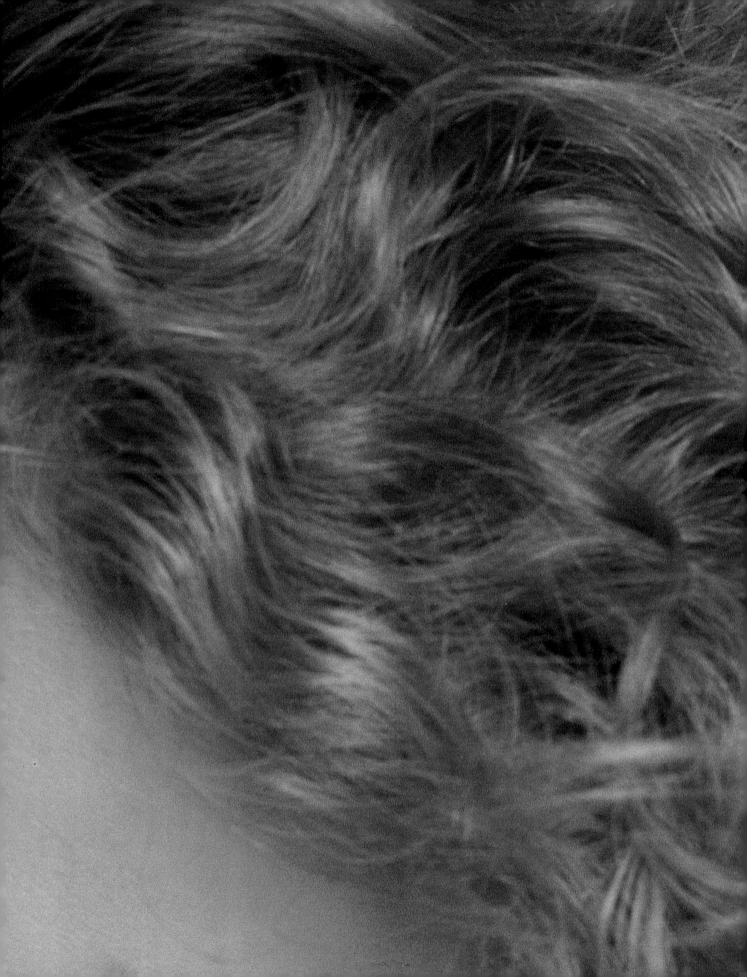

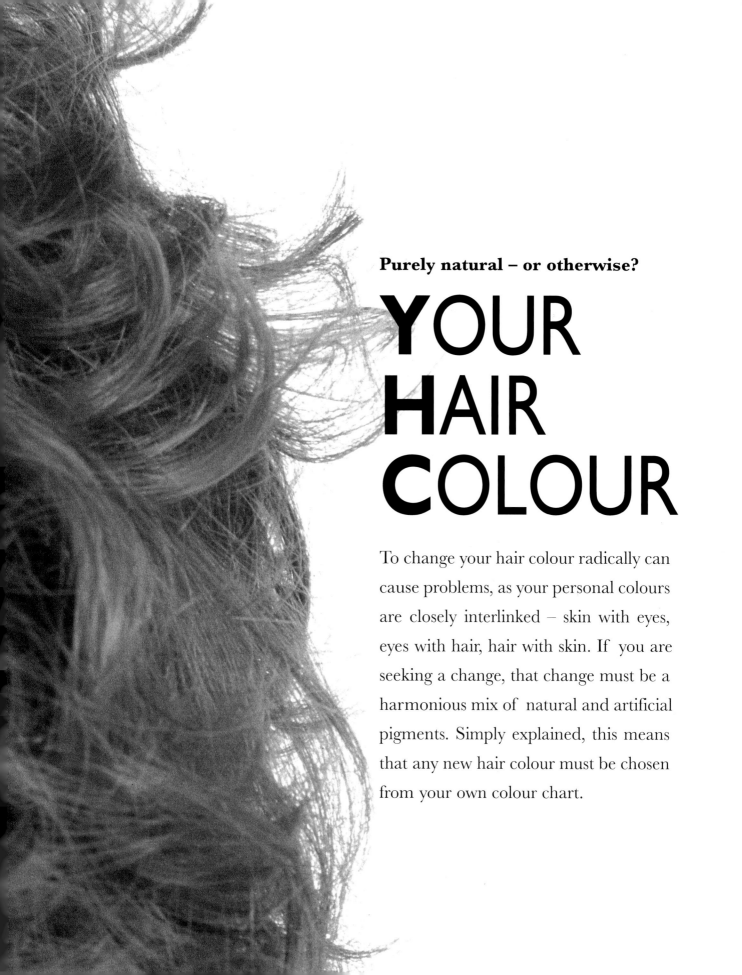

Purely natural – or otherwise?

YOUR HAIR COLOUR

To change your hair colour radically can cause problems, as your personal colours are closely interlinked – skin with eyes, eyes with hair, hair with skin. If you are seeking a change, that change must be a harmonious mix of natural and artificial pigments. Simply explained, this means that any new hair colour must be chosen from your own colour chart.

Is a colour change suitable for you?

To dye or not to dye? This is a difficult question. Some women automatically refuse to colour their hair because they are worried about how they will look and whether or not a new colour will suit them. So here's a thought: for many women their natural hair colour suits them best!

Other women may simply wish to experiment ... 'Do I look better, younger, more interesting if I change to a blonde, a redhead or a brunette? What about a few highlights?'

A professional colourist can colour your hair to any fashionable shade: it may be successful, it may not. But it can be fun to take a risk – your hair can be re-coloured if you don't like it and, of course, it will eventually grow out.

And, of course, a change can be good for you: hair is not just a frame for your face, but also a part of your identity. Who has not connected certain hair colours to personal traits – dark haired people are passionate, redheads are fiery, blondes are gentle and a brunette has a warm heart. As though it were that easy!

We are wrong to link character, mood and personality with hair colour.

Such assumptions still abound; they are easy to make and drop into a conversation. Indeed, a brunette may so wish to be thought of differently that she colours her natural, glossy rich hair a stark blue-black. Does it suit her? Another woman may bleach her hair white-blonde just because it is trendy and she wants to be noticed. And maybe this change will suit her. But should the experiment go badly wrong she will need the professional help of a good hairdresser to repair the hair while it grows back to its natural shade.

If you want to avoid making expensive, unpleasant mistakes, remember -

● If you are lightening your hair, the natural pigments are stripped from the hair shaft so that the new colour can be laid down instead. This process puts an incredible strain on to your hair which will continually need extra care and attention. Is it worth it?

● Anyone colouring their hair themselves regularly – and maybe using different brands and different colours – has no guarantee that they will achieve the desired result or that they will save money.

The results of successive colour changes are difficult to predict. If you are determined to make a colour change – particularly if a dramatic one – have it done by a professional (especially if something has already gone wrong with your own attempt).

If the hairdresser appears concerned that you have tried to colour your hair yourself, be patient. He knows his business.

The important point is the state of your hair – you are the customer, so pay for his good advice.

● Anyone wishing to add just a hint of colour to liven up their natural hair should try to determine what is their exact, natural shade before choosing their product. Remember, your hair may already be damaged by sea water and sun; the natural colour is found close to your scalp, at the back of your neck.

● A perm can also have an undesirable effect on hair colour! A hair's natural red pigment shows up more strongly when permed and increases in intensity as the hair is subjected to repeated chemical treatments. For Spring and Autumn types this isn't a problem as red, warm tones suit them well; in the case of the cooler Summer and Winter types however, this unexpected yellow red tint is unsuitable.

● If you are colouring your hair yourself use reputable products from well known manufacturers. Whether you use a shampoo, a cream or foam, a natural colour can easily be achieved and its intensity strengthened or lightened accordingly. But it is advisable not to use a home shampoo-in colouring product to bleach the hair. You should consider professional guidance if you require a dramatic, blonde look. And remember – if you don't like the new colour, it washes out very slowly over five or six shampoos.

● Highlights can be a very effective alternative. If you do not want to colour your hair totally and put your hair under such a strain, a few highlights around the face or on the crown are gently subtle. Whether you decide on intensive dyes or bleaches, a gentle wash-in colour tint, or only a few highlighted strands, what colour should you choose?

As you now know what colour season you belong to – Spring, Summer, Autumn or Winter – you should not be making any mistakes! There are just two simple rules to be observed.

Remember your colour chart – are you warm or cool? The wrong colour choice will clash with your complexion, and will make you appear tired and ungroomed. You can, of course, balance any mistake with cosmetics to enhance your new hair colour but this is time-consuming and could make you appear gaudy and brash.

And watch out for strong contrasts with your skin tone. Some women may look younger and fresher with the blonde hair of their childhood; for others a new blonde look could appear bland as their particular complexion needs a 'frame' of dark hair.

Other women could make the mistake of dyeing their hair too dark and instantly looking older. Why? The contrast is too hard for their complexion and the mix too ageing.

The choice of a lighter or darker hair colour is up to you. But always remember that the deciding factor is harmonisation – the new colour should harmonise with your complexion and eyes. Read the following pages to determine what is exactly right for you ...

The Spring type: soft and golden

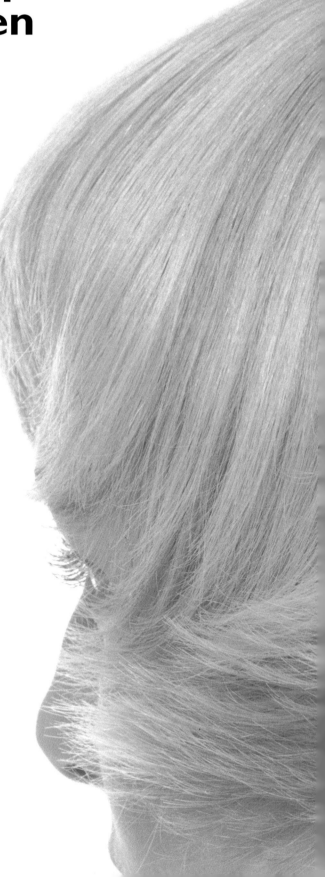

Most Spring types are naturally blonde with golden highlights. Others are lightly red. All Spring women should therefore remember that a strong, dramatic contrast is not for them – they mustn't destroy their natural delicacy. Many may find they already have natural highlights. If not, they could choose golden blonde and light copper highlights to liven up their hair. But remember – only warm tones suit a Spring woman's complexion. Silver blonde highlights could appear boring; sun yellow and honey colours such as warm red tones are best. As a fashionable alternative try a few highlights in bright, fiery orange. And who doesn't recall Marilyn Monroe's light Spring complexion looking fantastic with her bleached blonde hair!

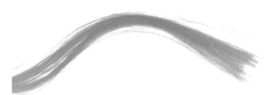

The warmer colours are ideal for the Spring woman; light blonde to make the hair lighter, copper or a golden dark blonde.

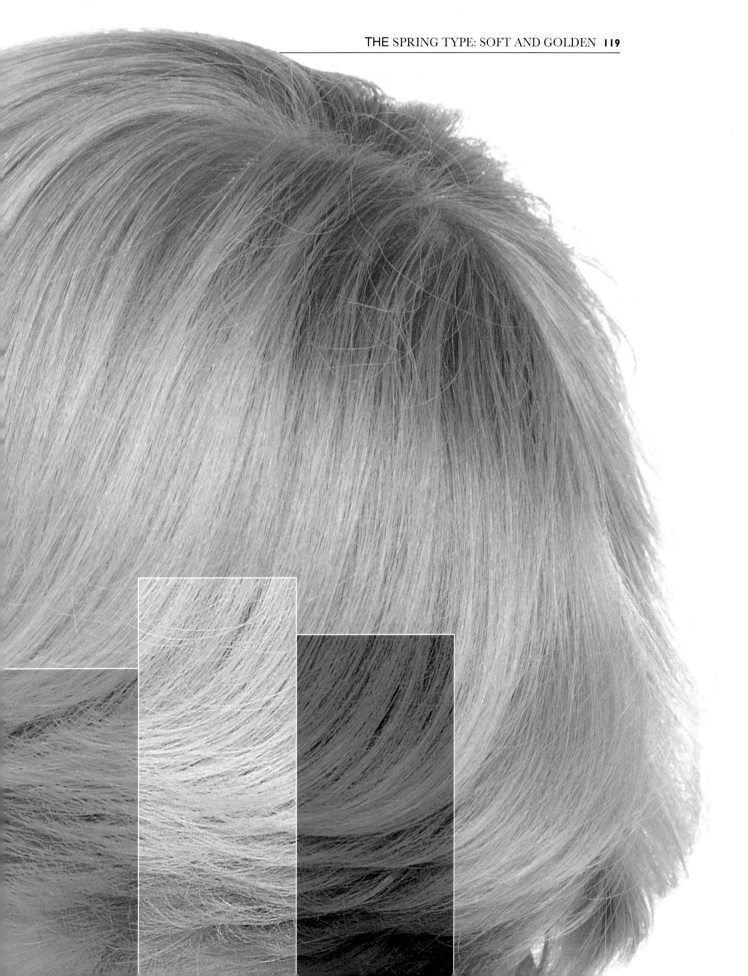

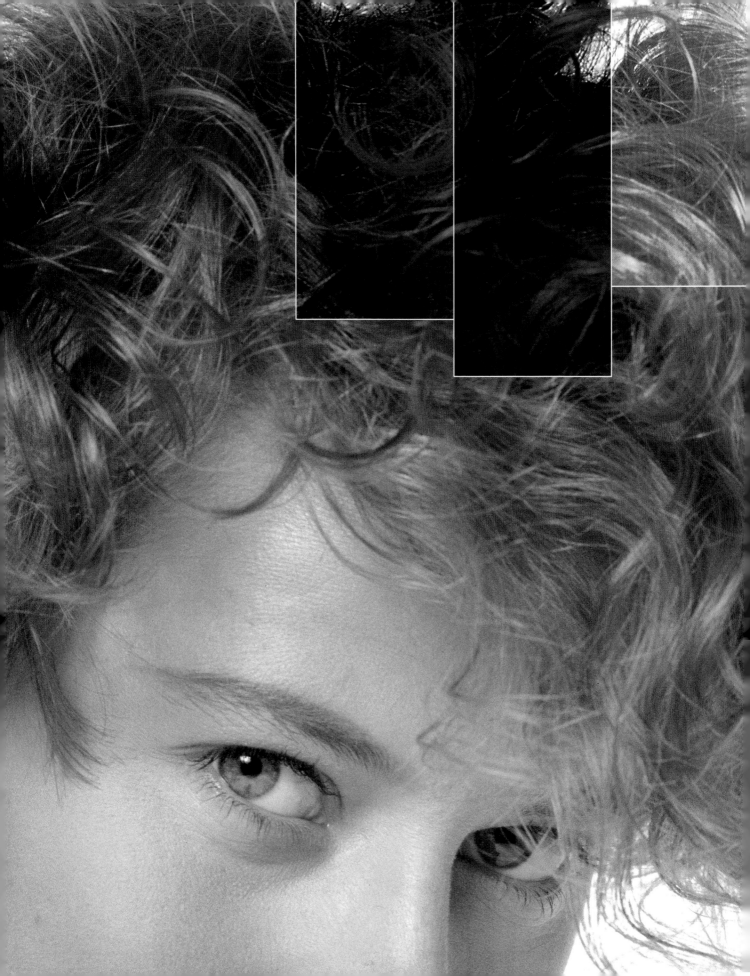

The Summer type: blonde to silver brown

Summer women can be unhappy with their hair colour. Not a glamorous blonde, dramatic black or exciting red, the Summer woman's hair is very often simply mousey. But with this as a base colour, the Summer woman is well placed to choose exciting colour options. Pretty, silver shimmering ash colours suit her intense complexion – this strengthens her natural colour. If a Summer woman decides to colour her hair red – which may actually suit some very well – then it must be a cool, bluish red shimmer, never a yellow orange! Summer women who had beautiful blonde hair as children look good with similarly blonde hair when older, livened with silver (not yellow) highlights. And don't forget platinum – some light-skinned Summer women look terrific with such an exciting colour mix.

Pale blonde highlights, cool mahoganies and deep ash blonde colours generally suit all Summer women – whatever their age. A fashionable tip: try a green highlight in ash blonde hair.

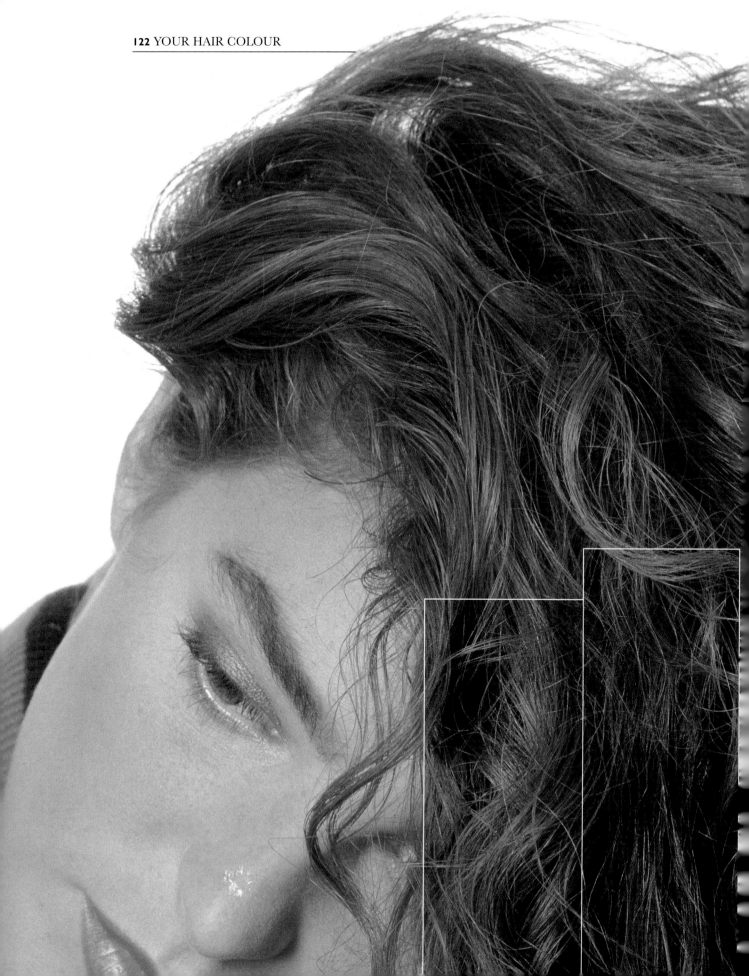

The Autumn: golden brown, red gold and deep brown

Imagine a light honey, a very dark forest amber and the many colours in-between – all perfect for the Autumn woman. Add to these colours a warm, golden shimmer or clear, fiery red; red blonde; coppery red; fox red; rust brown and chestnut brown. Autumn women with natural curls are advised not to lighten their hair as the process dries the hair and it will look frizzy and unmanageable. But many colour changes are possible including quite strong honey-blonde highlights that prettily display the curls. If their complexion is suitable, Autumn women with red hair can deepen their natural colour with a warm copper tone. And – as a cheeky, amusing accent – a fire red streak can look great (see below)!

Drastic changes are not for the Autumn woman. Depending on her base hair colour, she should consider all warm colours – from golden brown to dark copper.

The Winter type: natural is best

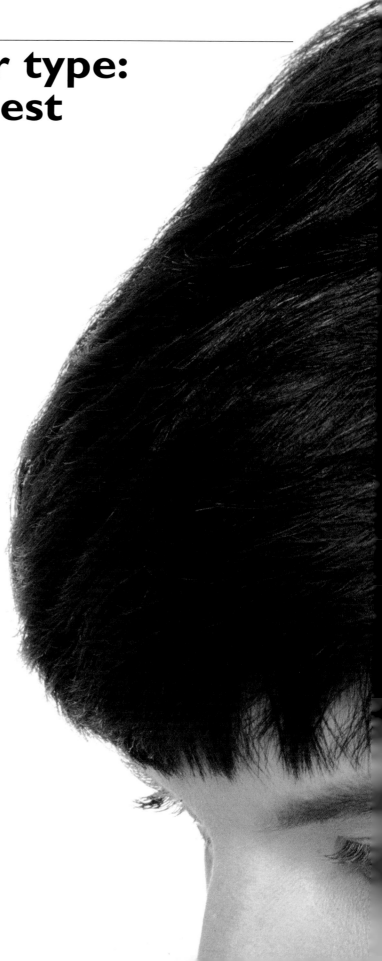

Winter women who like to experiment with colour will be disappointed with 'natural is best' but the best hairdresser will give the same advice.

With her dark hair and light skin colour contrast, the Winter woman looks very attractive naturally. A big change therefore would be a mistake. Even those few Winter women with blonde hair should be careful when bleaching their hair; every yellow tinge will make them look cheap instead of elegant. Brown haired Winter women should never try to turn themselves into Autumns with a warm red; it will not work.

The Winter woman suits cool colours – ash brown for a softer frame to their face, and blue-red for those women who have long admired redheads!

A fine violet streak is a fashionable trick for Winter women! Otherwise the Winter type shouldn't try too many experiments: only ash brown and the blue-red tones really suit her.

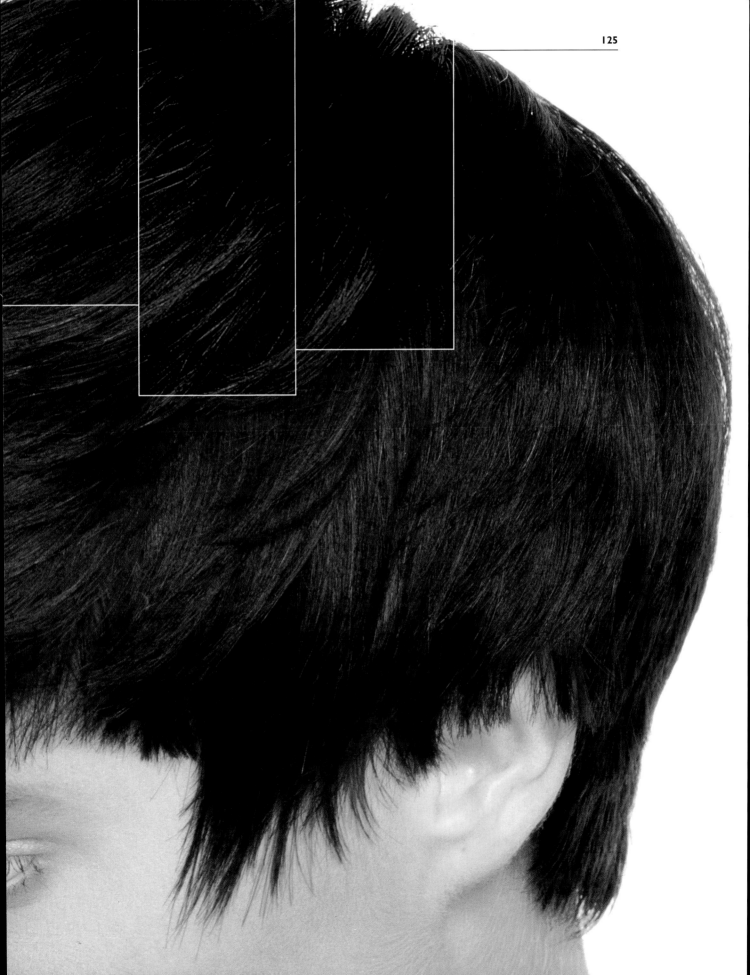

The secret of colours

Do you think you could live for any length of time in a brilliant, red painted room? Initially, you may find it exciting, but after a while it will disturb and disorientate you. Or imagine a clear, bright blue kitchen. Does it look clean and fresh? Yes, but without realising, you'll find yourself turning up the heating.

There are good reasons for talking about 'warm' and 'cool' colours. They have a strange effect on us and on the way we live our lives. For example, under scientifically controlled conditions, it is well known for people to misjudge the temperature of rooms painted in different colours. In warmly painted rooms, they feel warmer than the actual temperature and in rooms painted with cool colours, they shiver. Just imagination? Possibly, but the same research has suggested that even blind people can sense a difference ...

What is the answer? Maybe there isn't an immediate solution; maybe we feel colours instinctively, even magically. We do know that colour is nothing more than light reflected on a specific wavelength. The colour red has a different 'light' wavelength to that of blue; yellow a different one to violet and so on. Is this the secret?

There are 'warm' and 'cool' colours – we can feel the difference. Every living thing needs light to survive so why is it so surprising when we react to a particular colour? Why do we love some and not others? Why do some suit us and others don't? A simple colour test – tell me your favourite colour and I will tell you who you are, even which colour type you may be. There is little doubt; a sense of colour is a sense of self. A gentle rose-pink quietens anger – and this has been proved in family therapy and in prisons – being wrapped in a blue blanket soothes asthma sufferers and yellow is suggested for mental stimulation.

However, over time we all change – and our favourite colour can change according to our personality and our age.

Colours have long played a part in evolving cultures; they reflect our mood, calm us down or energise us. This is not a modern philosophy – the magic of colour has always been widely recognised. What is today's progressive 'colour therapy' is ancient knowledge: colours can help people live balanced and healthy lives.

Many different cultures have used colours to heal a damaged body and soothe an angry soul.

So which colours are your colours? Trust your instinct: you must know by now which colours suit you better than others. Take your time and decide which ones pacify you, which act as a tonic and which encourage you. One day you may prefer a dramatic red; the next a calmer blue-grey. In every single colour on your chart, you look good. But only you know which will suit you best from day to day.

INDEX

foulsham

The Publishing House, Bennetts Close,
Cippenham, Berkshire, SL1 5AP, England.

ISBN 0-572-02148-8

This edition copyright © 1996 W Foulsham & Co Ltd.
Originally published by Falken Verlag GmbH, 6272 Niedernhausen/Ts, Germany
in association with **freundin**
Photographs © Falken-Verlag.
Photographs supplied by: Otto Rauser
Contributors: Eberhard Henscher, Edda Kuffner, Rudi Gill, Thomas von Solomon,
Franziska Zingel, Villeroy & Boch, Micha Oxle, Horst Kirchberger, Michael Martin,
Ingeborg Wolff, Chilly Time, Jean Paul, Mayon, Mondi, Otto Keun, Pink Flamingo,
Portara, Virmani.
With thanks to Lady Manhattan Cosmetics, Schwarzkopf and Brendel Lunettes for
their friendly guidance and assistance in photographic production.

Printed in Great Britain by Cambus Litho, East Kilbride.